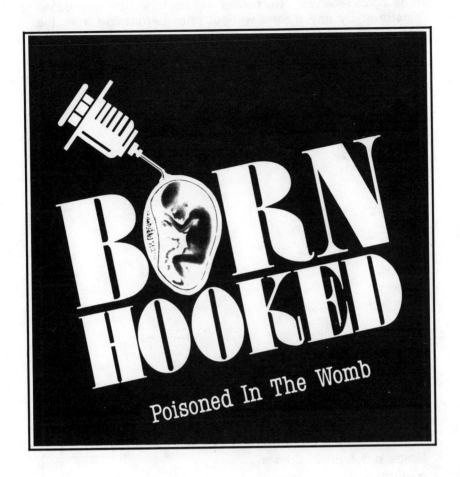

Gary E. McCuen

IDEAS IN CONFLICT SERIES

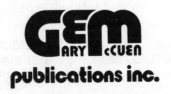

502 Second Street
Hudson, Wisconsin 54016

Illustrations & Photo Credits

David Seavey 12, 98, National Institute of Justice 16, 32, General Accounting Office 20, 76, 111, Craig MacIntosh 28, Engage/Social Action 38, 46, 51, 58, 67, 103, Bulletin of Municipal Foreign Policy 72, Locher 107, DEA Quarterly Intelligence Trends 115, Richard Wright 41. Cover illustration by Ron Swanson.

©1991 by Gary E. McCuen Publications, Inc.
502 Second Street, Hudson, Wisconsin 54016

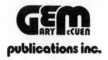

(715) 386-7113

International Standard Book Number 0-86596-080-1 Printed in the United States of America

CONTENTS

CHAPTER 4 FETAL NEGLECT AND
SOCIAL RESPONSE

CHAPTER 5 CRIME, PREGNANCY AND DRUGS

REASONING SKILL DEVELOPMENT

These activities may be used as individualized study guides for students in libraries and resource centers or as discussion catalysts in small group and classroom discussions.

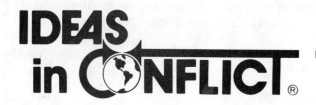

IDEAS in CONFLICT ®

This series features ideas in conflict on political, social, and moral issues. It presents counterpoints, debates, opinions, commentary, and analysis for use in libraries and classrooms. Each title in the series uses one or more of the following basic elements:

Introductions *that present an issue overview giving historic background and/or a description of the controversy.*

Counterpoints *and debates carefully chosen from publications, books, and position papers on the political right and left to help librarians and teachers respond to requests that treatment of public issues be fair and balanced.*

Symposiums *and forums that go beyond debates that can polarize and oversimplify. These present commentary from across the political spectrum that reflect how complex issues attract many shades of opinion.*

*A **global** emphasis with foreign perspectives and surveys on various moral questions and political issues that will help readers to place subject matter in a less culture-bound and ethnocentric frame of reference. In an ever-shrinking and interdependent world, understanding and cooperation are essential. Many issues are global in nature and can be effectively dealt with only by common efforts and international understanding.*

Reasoning skill *study guides and discussion activities provide ready-made tools for helping with critical reading and evaluation of content. The guides and activities deal with one or more of the following:*

RECOGNIZING AUTHOR'S POINT OF VIEW

INTERPRETING EDITORIAL CARTOONS

VALUES IN CONFLICT

WHAT IS EDITORIAL BIAS?

WHAT IS SEX BIAS?

WHAT IS POLITICAL BIAS?

WHAT IS ETHNOCENTRIC BIAS?

WHAT IS RACE BIAS?

WHAT IS RELIGIOUS BIAS?

From across **the political spectrum** *varied sources are presented for research projects and classroom discussions. Diverse opinions in the series come from magazines, newspapers, syndicated columnists, books, political speeches, foreign nations, and position papers by corporations and nonprofit institutions.*

About the Editor

Gary E. McCuen is an editor and publisher of anthologies for public libraries and curriculum materials for schools. Over the past years his publications have specialized in social, moral and political conflict. They include books, pamphlets, cassettes, tabloids, filmstrips and simulation games, many of them designed from his curriculums during 11 years of teaching junior and senior high school social studies. At present he is the editor and publisher of the *Ideas in Conflict* series and the *Editorial Forum* series.

CHAPTER 1

POISONED IN THE WOMB:
AN OVERVIEW

POISONED IN THE WOMB:
AN OVERVIEW

DRUG ADDICTED BABIES: A NATIONAL PERSPECTIVE

Ann K. Ruhmkorff

Drug and alcohol abuse in the United States is now recognized and acknowledged as a significant societal problem. The use of illicit drugs and alcohol occurs in all segments of the population, regardless of race, ethnicity or socioeconomic status. Drug use, especially cocaine, during pregnancy is no longer an unusual phenomenon. In fact, there has been an alarming increase in the last five years.

Statistics reported in 1987 indicated that five million people in the United States regularly use cocaine. This represents a five-fold increase in use during the past ten years. One in ten people have tried cocaine. Cocaine is the number one illicit drug used by women of childbearing age.

Alarming Statistics

A recent study by the National Association for Perinatal Addiction, Research and Education surveyed 36 hospitals across the country and found that at least 11% of women in the hospital have used illegal drugs during pregnancy. Ten to twenty percent of deliveries test positive for cocaine. The most alarming statistics were reported at a California conference on neonatal care and drug exposure, which stated an incidence of 18 to 21% positive drug screens in one local hospital.

Nationwide authorities estimate that approximately 400,000 babies annually are born addicted. Some physicians believe that as many as two-thirds of the children born with cocaine in their systems go undiscovered because hospitals do not routinely screen all newborns for drug levels.

Excerpted from a statement by Ann K. Ruhmkorff before the Subcommittee on Children, Family, Drugs and Alcoholism of the Senate Committee on Labor and Human Resources, October 9, 1989.

While cocaine is the drug most frequently associated with prenatal drug use, cocaine users typically use a combination of other drugs (Valium, opiates, amphetamines and marijuana) in addition to alcohol. It is extremely difficult to ascertain the frequency and amount of drug use during pregnancy.

Identifying Exposed Infants

The initial task of health care professionals is to identify drug-exposed infants. Withdrawal symptoms are well documented in infants born to heroin addicted mothers; however, there is some controversy concerning the presence of cocaine withdrawal symptoms. Whenever prenatal exposure to drugs is suspected, toxicology screens of both mother and infant should be performed. Common clinical signs of prenatal cocaine exposure include: hyperirritability, poor feeding patterns, abnormal suck and swallow, increased respiratory and heart rates, tremors, frequent startles and irregular sleeping patterns. These symptoms persist beyond the first few weeks of life and may be more indicative of central nervous system changes rather than a withdrawal pattern.

Cocaine addicted infants also have a higher rate of Sudden Infant Death Syndrome (SIDS), as much as 15% greater than the general population. These drug exposed infants are also at risk for a wide variety of medical complications, behavioral and developmental disabilities. Furthermore, these problems may become lifelong disabilities which may include: learning disabilities, slower intellectual development and delayed language development.

Of grave concern is the inability of the addicted infant to respond appropriately to his mother. The infant is unable to participate in interactive reciprocity, a component of the attaching process. To establish attachment (bonding), a newborn must respond in some way to the mother by initiating eye contact, grasping or cuddling. The newborn's behavior affects the resulting behavior of the mother. Studies have shown that the behavior of the newborn directly affects the caregiving he receives. In effect, a negative cycle may be set up in which the behavior of the poorly organized, irritable, high risk infant may suppress the optimal caregiving pattern necessary to facilitate his or her own recovery. The feeling of frustration and inadequacy that parents may experience in dealing with their fragile, yet unresponsive infant may predispose them later to physical child abuse.

Treatment Strategies

Health care professionals have developed interventions to enhance development of addicted infants and to decrease the atypical behavior patterns they exhibit. These include special positioning and handling strategies to decrease tremors, and feeding techniques that decrease oral defensiveness and normalize sucking behavior. Parent education is of paramount importance in enhancing normal infant development as well as ensuring a strong parent-infant bond. Parent education should begin as soon as possible, so that parents can learn appropriate and effective caregiving, Unfortunately, most drug dependent mothers have not had an adequate role model for parenting and therefore need to be taught basic parenting skills in addition to these special care techniques. It is important for parents to see the positive characteristics and strengths that their infant possesses, rather than focusing only on the weaknesses.

Without early intervention to normalize growth and development, there is an increased risk of creating a generation of children with long term learning disabilities and behavioral problems. The care of drug exposed infants requires committed caregivers (mother, relative or foster parent) who are willing to learn a practice of specific techniques of infant care and deal daily with an infant who is extremely irritable, difficult to feed and unresponsive to the caregiver's attempts at affection. This surely is not realistic for most drug dependent mothers, who suffer from low self-esteem and use drugs to escape from their problems. Discharging these infants from the hospital without a thorough assessment of the home environment, successful completion of a prenatal education program and active participation in an effective drug rehabilitation program may result in catastrophic injuries later in the child's life from abuse or lack of supervision. . .

Social Concerns

Unless all infants are tested for prenatal drug exposure, we may never know the scope of this problem, and we certainly will not be able to identify children at risk. Whether to indict and convict these mothers for exposing their child to drugs in utero is a difficult question to answer. If all mothers of drug exposed infants were prosecuted, our welfare system could not possibly

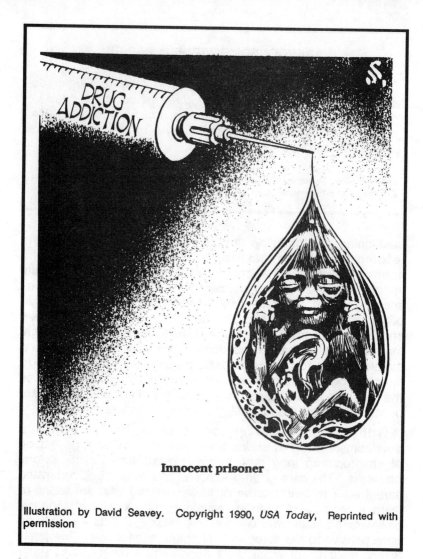

Innocent prisoner

Illustration by David Seavey. Copyright 1990, *USA Today*, Reprinted with permission

accommodate the demand for foster placement of these children. Marion County presently has a waiting list of 59 to 77 children weekly. With only 300 foster families presently available, the alternative for most of these infants would be placement in a group or residential homes. . .

The costs to society to care for drug exposed infants, abused children and catastrophic injuries related to parental drug use is staggering. In-patient hospital stays range from $500 to $1500 per day. Foster placement costs range from $8.50 to $25.00 per day. It seems that the money spent in prevention of maternal drug and alcohol abuse during pregnancy and drug rehabilitation programs after delivery would not only be more cost effective, but also may spare children from future abuse and injury.

POISONED IN THE WOMB:
AN OVERVIEW

PERINATAL DRUG ABUSE OCCURS IN ALL SOCIAL CLASSES

National Association for Perinatal Addiction, Research and Education (NAPARE)

The belief that problems associated with drug use by pregnant women occur primarily in lower socioeconomic, minority groups and not in the white middle class is erroneous, according to a new population-based study conducted by NAPARE and Operation PAR, Inc. in Pinellas County, Florida, for the Juvenile Welfare Board of the county.

Florida Study

Speaking to the national training forum on drugs, alcohol, pregnancy and parenting, held recently in Miami, Florida, Dr. Ira Chasnoff, who was the principle investigator, pointed out that the demographics of Pinellas County could be representative of many other communities across the United States. The county includes both urban (St. Petersburg and Clearwater) and suburban/ex-urban areas.

In the study, urine tests were conducted on every woman who enrolled for prenatal care at five Pinellas County public health clinics and every woman who entered similar care at 12 private obstetric practices in the county.

The study was conducted from January 1 to June 30, 1989. A total of 715 women were tested—380 in the clinics and 335 in private care. The tests were identified only by the patient's zip code, race and age.

Excerpted from "New Research Compares Drug Use by Public and Private Patients", *Update*, November, 1989, p.1. *Update* is the monthly newsletter of the National Association for Perinatal Addiction, Research and Education. (NAPARE)

Drugs and Infants

In Florida, a state-wide policy requires hospitals to notify the local health department when an infant is born with drugs in its system or the mother is addicted to or is abusing drugs or alcohol. Records from the Pinellas County health department during the same period were reviewed regarding all women who were reported for drug or alcohol abuse during pregnancy. Zip code, race and types of drugs consumed were recorded and compared with the statistics from the two groups of public and private patients.

The results showed:

14.8 percent of all the women tested positive for some drug(s) use—alcohol, marijuana, cocaine and/or opiates. There was no significant difference in the drug use rates of the private or public patients: 13.7 percent in the private sector and 16.3 percent in the public sector.

The incidence of the use of the individual drugs was also similar, except for cocaine having a slightly higher incidence among women in the public health group.

Among black and white women (both public and private patients), the rate of positive tests for drug use was 15 percent. Hispanic, oriental and Native American women were not included in these statistical analyses because of the small number in the study. The rate of positive tests for drugs among white women was 15.4 percent; the rate for black women, 14.1 percent.

In both the total population of women (public and private patients) and the total population of black and white women, marijuana was the drug used most often. In the total population of black and white women, black women showed a higher rate of cocaine use: 7.5 percent for black women, 1.8 percent for white women. White women used more marijuana: 14.4 percent versus 6 percent for black women.

In the six-month period of the study, 133 pregnant women were reported for substance abuse to the county health authorities: 48 were white; 85 were black. There were no significant differences in socioeconomic status, and patterns of drug use were similar.

In analyzing the proportion of women reported to the total number of births among black and white women, it was found that a black woman was 9.58 times as likely to be reported for substance abuse in pregnancy as compared to a white woman. This was in contrast to the fact that a white woman was 1.09 times as likely to have used drugs or alcohol just prior to her first prenatal visit to the doctor.

Explaining Preconceptions

Within the parameters of the study, no attempt was made to explain why the reporting difference existed. However, Dr. Chasnoff posed several hypotheses:

More white women may have stopped using drugs upon entering prenatal care, but other research indicates that drug use does not usually cease unless intensive therapeutic intervention is instituted.

Black infants may have demonstrated more severe symptoms of drug exposure, given that black women had a higher rate of cocaine use. While cocaine use can cause severe, obvious symptoms at birth that might lead physicians to test or attempt to take a drug use history, other research has demonstrated the impact of marijuana use on birth weight and neurobehavior and the existence of neurobehavioral changes in newborns exposed only to cocaine in the first trimester.

The preconception that substance abuse, especially during pregnancy, is a minority, urban, lower socioeconomic class problem may have biased physicians in their ascertainment of substance exposure in newborns.

Chasnoff challenged government bodies that are attempting to develop child protection laws which will cover substance abuse during pregnancy to be sure that medical evidence of drug use is the basis for determining risk and not preconceived notions of risk in certain populations.

He challenged health care professionals to examine personal biases that may influence lifestyle evaluations of their patients and diagnostic decisions.

Female Arrestees: Use of Cocaine*

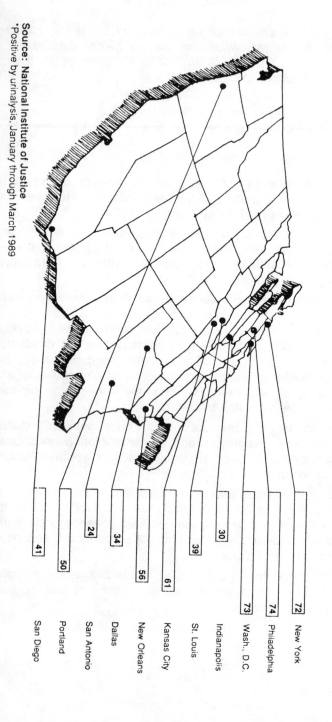

New York 72
Philadelphia 74
Wash., D.C. 73
Indianapolis 30
St. Louis 39
Kansas City 61
New Orleans 56
Dallas 34
San Antonio 24
Portland 50
San Diego 41

Source: National Institute of Justice
*Positive by urinalysis, January through March 1989

16

3

POISONED IN THE WOMB: AN OVERVIEW

IMPACT OF DRUGS ON INFANTS AND SOCIETY

Reed V. Tuckson

One area that I would like to focus my comments on in dealing with the total perspective of children and families is to focus on women, because that is really the key to what is happening with our children and our families as it relates to substance abuse in so many cases.

I attended a clinic in the poorest section of our city in southeast Congress Heights, and I remember vividly a pregnant woman who was an abuser of crack cocaine, and I asked her why she does this. As she talked to me about it, it became so very clear. She said, "I have no real sense of myself; I have no vision of the concept of the possibility of a meaningful future. I am not moving anywhere; I am caught, I am stagnant, I am not going anywhere. I am under-educated, I am unemployed, and I am really not building my life toward any sense of future or progress. I am caught in the moment. And so basically, she says, I do this to escape. I know it is wrong, but it is all around me."

Individuals and the Environment

"Living in this environment," she says, "living with the tensions, the pressures, the violence, the chaos, the family confusion, the dysfunctional people, I need something to get away from this." And I am very impressed and pleased that you focus on that as an issue because, as clinicians, we look for solving the causation of problems.

Reed V. Tuckson in testimony before the Senate Committee on the Judiciary, November 9, 1989. Mr. Tuckson is the Commissioner of Public Health for the District of Columbia.

When we look at the effect on the individuals and the women and the children in our community, we also have to look at what these drugs are doing to them physiologically and psychologically, particularly crack cocaine, which is the drug of choice now in our city and across urban, and really, national America—the extraordinary effects that we are seeing on the deterioration of heart functioning, the increase in heart rate, the extraordinary episodes of hypertension, the sudden death, as we witnessed tragically from another famous athlete, Len Bias.

We are very well aware of the increasing numbers of seizure disorders that we are seeing as we see the abnormal electrical activity in the brain, and then very dramatically, also, a decrease in the ability of the gastrointestinal tract to function, clamping off of the blood vessels there that causes people not to eat. And we see extremely malnourished, and thereby very vulnerable people whose immune systems don't work as well, who cannot ward off disease, who are not as productive.

Psychologically, we are seeing people, of course, who are addicted. We are seeing people who are depressed, anxious, irritable; people who are getting to the point now where there is a syndrome, a diagnosis called cocaine psychosis, an increasingly more common phenomenon.

Generally we are beginning to see the blunting of the human being, the blunting of the development and the growth and the maturation of the individual person, which concerns me greatly.

Increased Sexuality

There is an increased sexuality associated with this drug, not only because of the effects of the drug on sexual drive, but also increased sexuality in trade for the drug itself, selling your body to get the money or the drug to maintain the habit.

That is so tragic because now we see, despite the most unprecedented campaign in our country's history to avoid casual sexual experiences, to use a condom where appropriate all that education that is associated with AIDS—we now see a skyrocketing of sexually-transmitted diseases among the women of our community, among our entire community.

We know now that in 1985, our penicillin-resistant gonorrhea cases numbered 719; last year, 1,371. Syphilis cases in 1985 were 34 in this city; last year, 1,467. This is a direct result of the sexual activity and sexual behavior around the abuse of drugs—very, very important, and very frightening. And, of course, the HIV disease and the implications for that are obvious.

Sexual avtivity is not our only worry. We also find many people who are doing crack cocaine are now using heroin to come down from the effects of the cocaine. Even worse, many people are combining cocaine and heroin as a way to get an

18

added effect of the combination of drugs.

So 56 percent of the women in our community who have AIDS are I.V. drug users or drug abusers themselves, and the overwhelming majority of the remainder of those women are the sexual partners of drug abusers.

Problem Pregnancies

With increased sexuality, more people, of course, are pregnant. Then we have the problems with infant mortality, despite tremendous effort on the part of this city to bring down our infant mortality rate, which we were able to do in 1987, from 21 deaths per 1,000 in 1986 to 19.6 in 1987. That number has gone up to 23.2 last year, and all indications are that it will continue to go up this year directly as a consequence of substance abuse.

Every month in this city, the ambulances pick up at least 20 women who are pregnant and so compromised from the effects of these drugs that they require the services of our emergency medical system.

The babies that survive that process are children with speech and hearing deficits, learning disabilities, and/or anatomical malformations. As they grow older, we begin to see that these are babies that don't want to be held, that cry incessantly, that are irritable, that don't eat well, that don't retain their food, that have a plethora of other kinds of associated phenomena. These are children that are going to have very great problems in our society as they grow old, problems that this society is fundamentally unprepared to handle.

Finally, the other issue here is that these children too often are abandoned. They are left as boarder babies in our hospitals. We have now today 36 boarder babies in District of

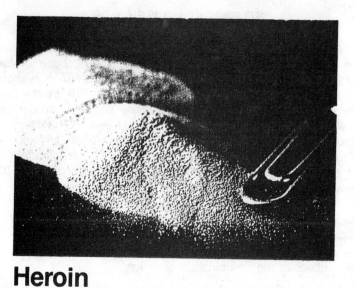

Heroin

Source: General Accounting Office

Columbia hospitals, 21 babies at D.C. General Hospital alone; a whole wing of babies. Five of those babies are HIV-positive.

Abuse and Neglect

We also know that there are increasing numbers of children being brought to us for child and family protective services as a result of abuse or neglect by women who are unable to manage their child care responsibilities. In fact, a child a day is brought to our system. We have 2,200 children currently in foster care in this city; 20 to 25 percent of the families in protective services are due to drug-related activity.

And I will conclude by saying that an even longer-term problem for us is that we find more and more grandmothers are now required to shoulder the responsibility of child-rearing when they have already paid their dues. They are already tired, they are already overloaded, and now they have got to manage much more complicated young people than they had to manage when they were, in fact, the primary care-givers in the past.

This is the range of challenges that confronts us. This is what we are seeing every day.

4

POISONED IN THE WOMB: AN OVERVIEW

DRUGS MOST COMMONLY ABUSED DURING PREGNANCY

NAPARE

Substances Most Commonly Abused During Pregnancy and Their Risks to Mother and Baby

When a pregnant woman drinks alcohol or abuses any drug, the developing fetus is also exposed to the harmful substance(s). These substances flow directly from the mother's bloodstream through the placenta and cross over to the baby. Harmful chemicals taken during the first three months of pregnancy can affect organ development or cause spontaneous abortion. Continued abuse may affect the baby's brain growth and weight gain or cause premature delivery.

Cocaine

During the first three months of pregnancy, there is an increased risk of spontaneous abortion. During the last three months, increased fetal movements and increased blood pressure and heart rate may occur. Intravenous cocaine abuse increases the risk of exposure to the AIDS virus. The newborn experiences withdrawal symptoms, and there is an increased risk of Sudden Infant Death Syndrome (SIDS-crib death).

Alcohol

Effects on the pregnant woman include malnutrition, increased risk of spontaneous abortion and increased rate of stillbirth. Effects on the baby include: Fetal Alcohol Syndrome (FAS), low birth weight, small head size, congenital malformations, withdrawal symptoms and behavioral problems, with possible mild to moderate mental retardation.

Excerpted from a paper by the National Association for Perinatal Addiction, Research and Education (NAPARE), 1989.

Heroin and Other Narcotics

Problems in the pregnant woman include hepatitis (both acute and chronic), endocarditis, spontaneous abortion, stillbirth and increased risk of contact with the AIDS virus if the substance is used intravenously. Problems in the infant include low birth weight and length, small head size, difficulty responding to the human voice and touch, withdrawal symptoms, and increased risk of SIDS (crib death).

Marijuana

Problems in the newborn include low birth weight, withdrawal symptoms and increased risk of SIDS.

The Dangers of Cocaine Use in Pregnancy

"Cocaine is popular, glamorous, middle-class, and plentiful — and possibly more dangerous to an unborn baby than any other illicit drug." Ira J. Chasnoff, M.D.

One in ten babies born in many urban areas of the United States has been exposed to cocaine in the womb according to research conducted at the Perinatal Center for Chemical Dependence at Northwestern Memorial Hospital, Chicago.

Many women believe the placenta acts as a shield but the opposite is true; it acts as a sponge. The characteristics of drugs that act on the central nervous system (mind-altering drugs) facilitate the passage of the drugs across the placenta from the maternal to the fetal circulation.

Even one use of cocaine during pregnancy puts the child at risk. Cocaine use during pregnancy puts the infant at least 10 times more at risk of Sudden Infant Death Syndrome (crib death).

Because cocaine acts as a stimulant to the central nervous system, causing constriction of blood vessels and rapid heart beat, the baby may suffer a sudden increase in blood pressure which results in acute infarction (stroke) while in the womb or shortly after birth.

The mother's intravenous drug use increases the risk of exposure to AIDS. Thirty to fifty percent of the infants born to HIV-positive mothers continue to test positive for the AIDS virus.

Cocaine use in the first trimester of pregnancy can cause spontaneous abortion or miscarriage. In the third trimester, cocaine use increases the risk of premature delivery.

Cocaine constricts the blood vessels in the placenta, cutting the flow of nutrients and oxygen to the fetus. Deformities and growth impairment may result. Drugs taken by the mother will remain longer in the fetus than in the adult because of the immaturity of the fetal liver.

Infants of mothers who use cocaine tend to have lower birth weights and to be shorter and have smaller head circumferences than infants delivered to a drug-free women.

Cocaine addicted infants have more of a psychological than a physical problem with withdrawal. An exposed baby remains irritable for six to eight weeks after birth and doesn't respond well to its environment for two or three months. The mother may be less likely to provide the needed comfort and nurturing to an irritable and unpredictable baby, so its psychological development is hampered.

Cocaine addicted babies account for 80 percent of the drug—affected babies born to women who are participating in the program at Northwestern Memorial Hospital's Perinatal Center for Chemical Dependence.

CHAPTER 2

COCAINE BABIES

COCAINE BABIES

A NEW BIO-UNDERCLASS

Charles Krauthammer

Charles Krauthammer is a nationally syndicated political columnist. He also writes weekly for The New Republic *magazine.*

Points to Consider:

1. What is meant by the phrase, "a bio-underclass"?

2. How serious is the problem of cocaine babies?

3. Identify the damage infants can suffer from a cocaine pregnancy.

4. How is the problem of cocaine babies compared to the "Brave New World" of Aldous Huxley?

A cohort of babies is now being born whose future is closed to them from day one.

The inner-city crack epidemic is now giving birth to the newest horror: a bio-underclass, a generation of physically damaged cocaine babies whose biological inferiority is stamped at birth.

"This is not stuff that Head Start can fix," explains Douglas Besharov, former director of the National Center on Child Abuse who coined the term bio-underclass. "This is permanent brain damage. Whether it is 5 percent or 15 percent of the black community, it is there. And for those children it is irrevocable."

An estimated 5 percent of New York City infants are exposed to cocaine in the womb. In the District of Columbia, it is 15 percent. Although this catastrophe is particularly acute in the black community, it is obviously not restricted to it.

Besharov estimates that one-half of 1 percent of all babies born in the United States have been exposed to cocaine. Throughout the country the problem is exploding. In 1985, two cocaine babies were born in Cincinnati. This year, University Hospital there expects 120.

Crack

Crack accounts for the astonishing jump in infant mortality rates in places like the District of Columbia. Cocaine babies have 15 times the risk of Sudden Infant Death Syndrome. But the dead babies may be the lucky ones.

For some of the crack babies who survive, the first life experience is the agony of cocaine withdrawal. They suffer terribly. They are so sensitive to touch that they cannot be held or fed properly. Some move their limbs endlessly, looking for relief.

Even hardened veterans of intensive care units find the high pitched cries of withdrawing babies intolerable. "Never in my medical career have I seen so much suffering as cocaine has brought," says the director of the nursery at D.C. General Hospital.

Appalling Damage

A mother's use of cocaine during pregnancy can cause appalling damage to the infant: strokes, seizures, paralysis, prematurity, deformed hearts and lungs, abnormal genital and intestinal organs, and, most ominously, permanent brain damage.

A cohort of babies is now being born whose future is closed to them from day one. Theirs will be a life of certain suffering, of probable deviance, of permanent inferiority. At best, a menial life of severe deprivation; at worst, early and painful death all biologically determined from birth.

Brave New World

It is a horror worthy of Aldous Huxley. In *Brave New World* the state creates a race of subhuman "Epsilon" drones by reducing their oxygen as they incubate in government-run fetal "hatcheries." "Nothing like oxygen-shortage for keeping an embryo below par," explains Mr. Foster, a hatchery scientist, rubbing his hands.

Cocaine works the same way. It does its damage in the womb by cutting off the blood supply to the baby, leaving every organ, the brain in particular, screaming for oxygen.

Yet life has outdone Huxley. Even he could only imagine a mad utopian state doing this to its children. It is harder to imagine mothers doing it to their own. Yet, says Dependency Court Commissioner Stanley Genser of Los Angeles County, "We are getting women in here now who have given birth to their second or third or fourth drug baby."

Indians

It is not just in the inner city that a bio-underclass is emerging. Alcohol is creating a similar bio-underclass among Indians. Studies show that on some reservations 5 to 25 percent of children suffer from fetal alcohol syndrome, physical abnormalities and mental retardation caused by heavy maternal drinking during pregnancy. The children are hyperactive, difficult to raise, harder to educate. They have been robbed of the capacity for thinking well. The consequence, pediatrician Geoffrey Robinson says, is "a devastation that is worse than

27

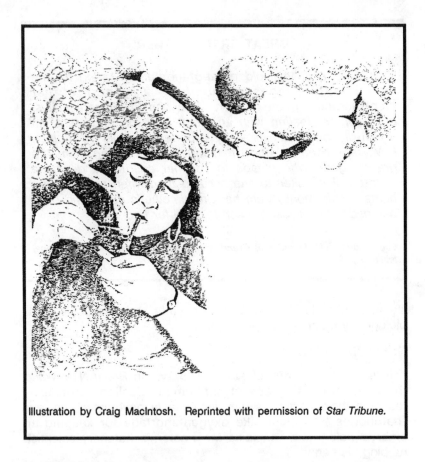

Illustration by Craig MacIntosh. Reprinted with permission of *Star Tribune*.

smallpox."

Maternal drug and alcohol abuse is producing damaged babies throughout society. A 1985 survey by the National Institute on Drug Abuse found that at least one in 10 of all American women of childbearing age had used cocaine in the previous year. The problem exists among the middle class, although middle class money can at least help protect these children after birth.

Menace to Future

When the problem becomes concentrated and localized, as in the inner city or on the reservation, it becomes a threat to communal life as a whole. In the poorest, most desperate pockets of American society, it has now become a menace to the future.

For the bio-underclass, the biologically determined underclass of the underclass, tomorrow's misery will exceed yesterday's. That has already been decreed.

COCAINE BABIES

POISONED BABIES IN THE NATION'S CAPITOL

Margaret L. Gallen

Margaret L. Gallen, CNM, MSN, has been a Registered Nurse since 1953 and a Certified Nurse Midwife since 1969. Her entire professional experience has been in the area of Maternal and Child Health both in the United States and in Africa. She has been the Director of the Nurse Midwifery Service at D.C. General Hospital since 1975.

Points to Consider:

1. Describe the "raw" statistics on pregnant mothers who use drugs.

2. What evidence of drug use is presented?

3. Why is cocaine a damaging drug?

4. Why are more pregnant women using crack-cocaine?

Margaret L. Gallen in testimony before the House Select Committee on Children, Youth, and Families, April 24, 1989.

Women are using sex to pay for their crack, and in their desperation there is little thought given to safer or responsible sex.

D.C. General Hospital is located at 19th & Mass. Ave., S.E., literally a "stones' throw" from the Capitol Building. It shares a twenty-six acre campus with the D.C. Jail, and D.C. Department of Human Services out-patient and in-patient substance abuse facilities, a mental health clinic, sexually transmitted disease clinic and tuberculosis clinic. Our metro stop has been named "Stadium-Armory" though I can't imagine why, as those facilities function only occasionally and our campus almost explodes with activity daily.

Growing Concern

I realize that throughout the entire nation, there is a growing concern about chemical substance abuse and its attendant ills, including increased violence, crime, child abuse and maternal and newborn sickness and death. Let me tell you how this plays out in Washington, D.C. in 1989.

First, a review of even very "raw" statistics shows that in the months of January, February and March of 1987 one mother of every ten coming into our Admissions Office in labor responded positively to the physician's question, "Are you using any drugs?" For January, February and March of 1989 one mother in five answered "yes". To date, this month has shown a one percent increase over the previous three months. How many other mothers decline to answer truthfully we do not know, as a Toxicology Screen is not a part of routine laboratory tests gathered but is performed with the patient's knowledge only if signs or symptoms of substance abuse exist.

Daily Events

Numbers alone cannot give you the full picture of what is now becoming an almost daily occurrence: that of a woman pregnant, "high" on drugs with extreme anxiety for her own and her baby's life stating that she has lost control of her own ability to resist the compulsion to smoke crack. She comes literally begging the hospital to admit her to the Obstetrical Unit to protect her from herself. Consider the following scenarios which have all occurred since January and show so well some other evidence of usage.

a. A twenty-two year old prenatal substance abuser in the midst of a discussion of treatment for a sexually transmitted disease, tears up her medical record and leaves without treatment thus continuing to expose her baby and sexual partners.

30

b. A twenty-five year old woman is admitted unconscious, in labor with a history of seizures while at home. Her urine toxicology is positive for cocaine and she wakes up three days after delivery asking to eat.

c. A pregnant thirteen year old, incarcerated in the City's Receiving Home, is brought to the Obstetrics and Gynecology Department at D.C. General. Allegedly, she is in custody for transporting crack from New York to Washington.

d. A twenty-eight year old mother comes into the hospital by ambulance with a four pound eight ounce dead male newborn and placenta, claiming she last free based cocaine three days prior to delivery.

e. A thirty-eight year old pregnant woman comes to the hospital by ambulance having seizures, semi-comatose but still clinging to a piece of crack. A live infant is delivered by emergency cesarean section, but the mother dies while still in the delivery room.

f. A mother comes into the hospital in labor carrying a revolver for her own protection and saying someone is out to get her. The gun is confiscated by the Metropolitan Police and she spends her hospitalization accompanied by a policewoman. This demonstrates the extent of the violence in Washington, D.C.

g. Our adolescent mothers present a new problem because

31

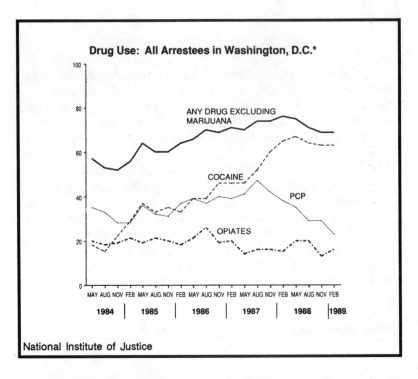

Drug Use: All Arrestees in Washington, D.C.*

ANY DRUG EXCLUDING MARIJUANA

COCAINE

PCP

OPIATES

National Institute of Justice

frequently their families are now unable to be as supportive as they might have been and must be, if the young unexperienced mother is to be successful as a parent. . .

h. We have had young mothers who cannot take their babies home to their own mothers because the home has turned into a "crack house". . .

i. The D.C. jail has numerous young mothers and expectant mothers within its population. . .The women are quite open in discussing the intensity of the addiction and the rapidity with which a person loses control over her life. Recently a woman described how her neighbor sold her baby to someone just to get enough money to satisfy her compulsion.

j. Recently we have heard of instances where women, knowing that it causes irritation of the uterus, have purposely taken crack to induce labor or to effect a speedy labor. A mother at the jail described how she delivered a nine and a half pound baby in an hour while under the influence of crack.

I realize that this all sounds melodramatic but it only illustrates how the chemical changes induced by crack-cocaine on the brain have pervaded and poisoned the total community. Why is my continuous referral to crack-cocaine rather than to heroin or PCP? Because crack is now the "drug of choice" in the District and even those who have been using heroin for years are now

32

also smoking crack as it provides the ultimate "high". Authorities report that PCP used alone is fast becoming a rarity. Most now use PCP and crack together to achieve a more gradual "low". Crack itself is often smoked with marijuana.

Damaging Drug?

What makes this drug and its route of administration so damaging? Basically you should remember that crack is a highly concentrated form of cocaine: that it costs far less than the traditional "avant-garde" form of cocaine, hydrochloride, thus making it within the reach of even the most modest pocketbook; that it causes in laboratory animals observable and reproducible changes in brain chemistry which make addiction almost a certainty; that by smoking crack-cocaine rather than snorting it, the desired effect is almost instantaneously achieved but wears off very quickly, thus necessitating the use of more drugs very quickly. . .

Problem in Pregnancy

What makes crack usage such a problem in pregnancy? First, you need to know that when a woman is pregnant her metabolism increases considerably because she really is breathing for two, eating for two, voiding for two, etc., even to the point that the mother's thyroid gland is enlarged. Now you add crack which in a matter of seconds makes all her blood vessels constrict, makes her blood pressure literally shoot up, and her heart beat so fast she will tell you that it feels as though it's about to jump out of her chest, you can imagine what this does to an already overloaded system. Too, in normal circumstances there is more than a pint of blood going to the maternal uterus each minute where it is to deliver oxygen to the baby and take away his carbon dioxide. With such constriction of the mother's blood vessels, the blood supply is decreased; the baby does not get an adequate supply of oxygen, and slowly but surely the carbon dioxide builds up in his body because it can't be taken away fast enough. The real emergency comes when the pressure in the mother's blood vessels becomes so high that it is able to force the afterbirth off the wall of the uterus.

More Pregnant Crack Users

Why do we have so many more women pregnant when using crack than we had in years past with heroin-using women? Simple, the women are using sex to pay for their crack and in their desperation there is little thought given to safer or responsible sex. As a result we are now seeing more addicted pregnant women but we are also seeing an increase in sexually transmitted diseases throughout the community. Incidentally, more and more frequently we are also noting that the germs causing these sexually transmitted diseases (STD) are resistant to the "miracle drugs" we once thought were going to solve all of our venereal disease problems. . .

What assessment can we make after my depressing review of the crack-cocaine problem?

a. This is not an epidemic; it is a pandemic.

b. Maternal and infant morbidity and mortality (sickness and death) statistics for the United States will surely rise in the near future.

c. AIDS in the heterosexual, non-IV drug-abusing population will surely rise in the near future.

d. Gynecological cancer rates will surely rise in the near future as certain other types of viruses are passed around.

e. We do not have too much more time left for discussion when you realize that it has been estimated that ninety percent of crack users become addicted, and that from first "high" till the person "hits bottom" can take as little as six months.

f. The effect on the school systems across this nation in the next few years can only be imagined as they are challenged by an increase in the numbers of socially and physically impaired children.

g. Metropolitan areas which have been hit the hardest need HELP, HELP, HELP.

COCAINE BABIES

FETAL DRUG ABUSE: THE NATIONAL PROBLEM

Neal Halfon

Neal Halfon, M.D., M.P.H. is the director of the Center for the Vulnerable Child Ambulatory Services at Children's Hospital in Oakland, California. He is also Assistant Clinical Professor of Pediatrics and Health Policy in the Department of Pediatrics and Institute for Health Policy Studies at the University of California in San Francisco.

Points to Consider:

1. How is the prevalence of drug exposure to babies in utero described?

2. Describe the medical costs of drug-addicted babies.

3. What are the pre- and post-natal effects of intrauterine drug exposure?

Neal Halfon in testimony before the House Select Committee on Children, Youth and Families, April 24, 1989.

A profile of pregnant women who use crack-cocaine reveals that they have been victims of physical, sexual, and emotional abuse as children and adults.

Ira Chasnoff, M.D., of Northwestern University, surveyed 36 hospitals across the country (accounting for 150,000 births) and showed that 11% of births had positive toxicological screens for illicit drugs. . .

A prospective study conducted by Barry Zuckerman, M.D., and published in the March, 1989, *New England Journal of Medicine,* indicated that 18% of all births at Boston City Hospital demonstrated cocaine exposure. . .

A survey in Oakland in 1988 reported that 16% of all births at Highland General Hospital were positive for cocaine.

Most urban hospitals in California now report that between 10 and 20% of all births show evidence of drug exposure. . .

Estimates would suggest that almost 30,500 babies exposed to drugs will be born this year in California. Until more accurate surveillance is undertaken, these estimates will be only ballpark approximations. It should be noted that the 30,500 figure for California is consistent with Chasnoff's estimate that 375,000 babies will be born drug-exposed this year in the United States.

Prenatal Effects

Cocaine and its metabolites increase the heart rate and blood pressure of the mother and decrease the supply of oxygen to the fetus through constriction of the blood supply to the placenta. Cocaine also is a strong appetite suppressant and can decrease essential weight gain, potentially hampering fetal nutrition. . .

A Chicago study indicates that babies of women who, because of intervention, use cocaine only during the first trimester do not necessarily escape all ill effects, but do display lower levels of prematurity and abruption, and no intrauterine growth retardation. The implications of the study are that early intervention and cessation of crack-cocaine use in the first trimester can lessen many of the drug's effects and prevent other long term complications.

Postnatal Effects

Data are available on cocaine's effects on the first year of life, to a lesser extent on toddlers, and, to a much lesser extent, on preschool and school-aged children.

In infancy we find:

— irritability and hypersensitivity

— movement disorders and increased stiffness

- fine motor deficits
- increased incidence of Sudden Infant Death Syndrome (SIDS)

Toddlers exposed to crack often:

- are irritable and display poor impulse control and less goal-directed behavior
- are less securely attached to caretaker
- are distracted and easily frustrated
- have expressive language difficulties
- demonstrate less free play
- lack ability to self-regulate

Preschool-aged children demonstrate:

- learning difficulties
- language problems
- continuation of toddler problems

School-aged children, about whom relatively little is known, appear to show persistent cognitive and emotional delays.

The Maternal and Family Context of Chemical Dependency and Exposure

A profile of pregnant women who use crack-cocaine reveals that:

- they have been victims of physical, sexual, and emotional abuse as children and adults;
- drug use has become an unsuccessful coping style to deal with persistent exposure to violence including physical abuse and rape;
- a majority were raised in homes where one or both parents used drugs and/or alcohol;

37

- they are likely to live with a drug using partner and are often subjected to physical violence in these relationships;
- they need but have often been unsuccessful in receiving treatment for their chemical dependency and for both their biological and psychological signs and symptoms;
- they need housing, food, job training and education;
- they do not have access to or avail themselves of prenatal care;
- they have an increased prevalence of other medical and psychological problems including low self-esteem and social isolation;
- they are at increased risk for HIV infections secondary to IV drug use, prostitution and exchange of sex for drugs;
- they are at increased risk for other sexually transmitted diseases including syphilis, hepatitis B, and herpes. . .

Even given all the difficulties and potential problems, well designed comprehensive programs can provide mothers with resources to overcome their drug addiction illness and become adequate parents.

Impact on Foster Care System

Many drug-exposed babies are placed into foster care at birth or in the first years of life. In some cases as many as 60% of drug-exposed babies go into foster care. Recent studies report that increases in drug use are mirrored by statewide increases in the number of children entering the foster care system. . .

This flooding of the foster care system has important ramifications for a system which was already overburdened and lacking sufficient resources. For example, from 1986 to 1988, the average stay in foster care increased 30 percent, from 15 months in 1986 to 20 months in 1988.

We also know that the foster child population has become younger, largely as a result of perinatal drug exposure and placement soon after birth.

Cost for Perinatal Health Services

Because of the prenatal effects of drug exposure and the fact that nearly 30 percent of infants exposed in utero are born premature, the increased costs in perinatal health services are dramatic:

In Los Angeles County, 915 infants born in 1986 were estimated to cost $32 million because of extended hospital stays.

70% were term babies, hospitalized on average for 9 days, at $600/day, or $5,400/child.

38

12% were premature babies with uncomplicated courses hospitalized on average for 42 days, at $1500/day, or $63,000/child.

18% born premature with complications were hospitalized on average for 90 days, at $1,500/day, or $135,000/child.

Similar but smaller numbers are seen in Alameda County where in 1987, 48 severely ill premature babies born in Alameda County were transferred to the Neonatal Intensive Care Unit (NICU) at Children's Hospital in Oakland with an average length of stay of 41 days, totaling 1,986 NICU days, at an estimated cost of $2.6 million.

Rough estimates can be generated of the potential hospital cost for a projected population of 30,000 drug-exposed infants born in California each year (roughly 5% of all births). Using the cost generated from the Los Angeles County study, assuming a prematurity rate of 30%, the cost for perinatal hospital care would exceed $1 billion. Since the rate of prematurity in some poor communities approaches 15%, this excess of 15% prematurity still would account for $500 million of hospital expenditures per year.

Interpreting Editorial Cartoons

This activity may be used as an individualized study guide for students in libraries and resource centers or as a discussion catalyst in small group and classroom discussions.

Although cartoons are usually humorous, the main intent of most political cartoonists is not to entertain. Cartoons express serious social comment about important issues. Using a graphic and visual format, cartoonists may have as much or more impact on national and world issues as editorial and syndicated columnists.

Points to Consider:

1. Examine the cartoon in this activity. (see next page)

2. How would you describe the message of the cartoon? Try to describe the message in one to three sentences.

3. Do you agree with the message expressed in the cartoon? Why or why not?

4. Does the cartoon support the author's point of view in any of the readings in this publication? If the answer is yes, be specific about which reading or readings and why.

5. Are any of the readings in Chapter Two in basic agreement with the cartoon?

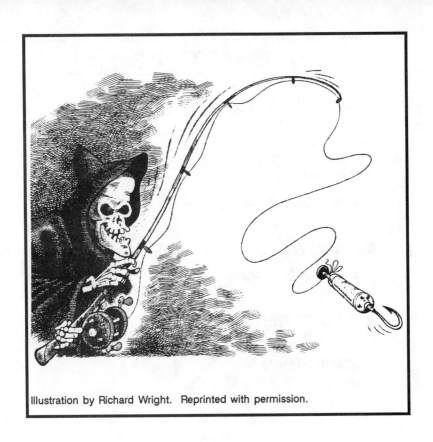

Illustration by Richard Wright. Reprinted with permission.

CHAPTER 3

FETAL ALCOHOL SYNDROME

8   FETAL ALCOHOL SYNDROME

ALCOHOL AND BIRTH DEFECTS: AN OVERVIEW

U.S. Public Health Service

The following statement was reprinted from a public paper released by the U.S. Public Health Service. The statement describes relation-ships between alcohol and birth defects.

Points to Consider:

1. What is Fetal Alcohol Syndrome (FAS)?

2. How prevalent is FAS?

3. Identify deformities seen in babies with FAS.

4. Explain the effects of low level drinking on fetuses during pregnancy.

U.S. Public Health Service, " Alcohol and Birth Defects," printed 1988.

Gross deformities seen in babies with FAS are most conspicuous in the eyes, midface, and cranium.

It is now widely accepted by medical authorities and researchers that women who drink during pregnancy can adversely affect the development of their unborn infants. The Fetal Alcohol Syndrome (FAS), first described by researchers in France in 1968 and corroborated by American researchers in 1973, is the most severe form of alcohol-induced malformation and is seen only in the infants of severely alcoholic women who drank heavily throughout pregnancy. Hundreds of case reports of FAS have been published since the syndrome was first recognized. There have also been numerous reports of partial manifestations of FAS in the offspring of women who drank substantial amounts of alcohol during pregnancy but at less than alcoholic levels. Finally, there is evidence that subtle behavioral effects may occur in the offspring of women who drink at moderate or "social" levels during pregnancy. Thus it appears that the effects of drinking during pregnancy lie on a continuum. The effects can range from severe to subtle, depending on the amount of alcohol consumed during pregnancy.

The Fetal Alcohol Syndrome

Gross deformities seen in babies with FAS are most conspicuous in the eyes, midface, and cranium. They include small eye openings, drooping eyelids, small eyes, skin folds across the inner corners of the eyes (abnormal in Caucasians), a flattened or missing bridge of the nose, underdeveloped philtrum (the depression in the skin between the nose and upper lip), thin upper lip, an exaggerated space between the nose and upper lip, and small head circumference. In addition, there is mental retardation ranging from serious to profound. The children never outgrow these handicaps, as shown by followup studies extending into the teen years.

Prevalence of FAS

Although there are no firm data on the prevalence of FAS, estimates have been obtained by several studies in the United States and Europe. A generally accepted estimate of FAS prevalence based on these studies is one to three cases of FAS per 1,000 live births. However, recent evidence indicates that some racial and cultural groups—blacks and certain American Indian groups, for example—are at greater risk of FAS than the population as a whole.

An extremely high rate of FAS has been reported in certain American Indian populations in the Southwest. A study in 1982-1983, comparing FAS prevalence in a population sample of about 240,000 representing three Indian cultural groups, found

FAS prevalence to be within the general population estimates among the Navajo and Pueblo cultures, as well as among Southwestern Indians in general. However, in certain areas the rate of FAS was extremely high—9.8 cases of FAS per 1,000 births, or about one percent of all live births. The reason for the extraordinary prevalence is not known, although genetic susceptibility, type of beverage customarily consumed, and cultural patterns regarding alcohol use could all be involved.

What Determines Susceptibility to Prenatal Alcohol Damage?

Not all women who drink abusively during pregnancy deliver babies with FAS or alcohol-related birth defects. The frequency of these alcohol-related birth anomalies is, in fact, much lower than the frequency of heavy drinking among pregnant women. It would appear, then, that other factors operate to modify the risk of prenatal alcohol damage. What these other factors may be is a question that is only beginning to be explored systematically.

A recent epidemiological study involving examination of data on 5,093 pregnant women in Loma Linda, California, and 8,331 pregnant women in Cleveland found that beverage type plays a significant role in modifying the risk of fetal alcohol damage. Although it is well demonstrated that any kind of alcoholic beverage consumed during pregnancy can cause birth defects, beer, for unknown reasons, was found to pose a higher risk.

Factors adding significantly to the risk of alcohol-induced birth defects were increased maternal age, previous history of alcohol problems, greater proportion of drinking days during pregnancy, higher proportion of alcohol from beer, and black race. If all these factors were present, the probability of an FAS baby being born to a drinking mother was more than 50 times greater than if none were present. Black race alone was found to increase

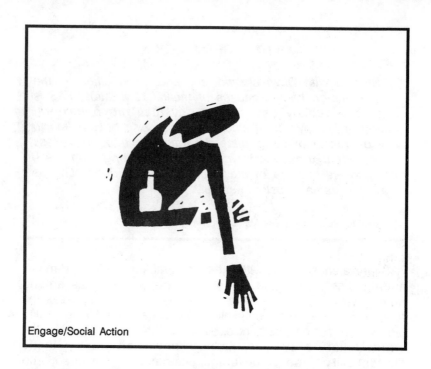

Engage/Social Action

the risk for FAS to a level about seven times higher than for white infants who received the same prenatal alcohol exposure.

Although these studies indicate that race may be an important factor affecting risk for FAS, it is important to note that numerous studies around the world have demonstrated that no racial or ethnic group is immune.

Effects of Lower Levels of Drinking During Pregnancy

Hundreds of case reports from many nations indicate that the full FAS is seen only in the children of women who were alcoholics and drank heavily throughout their pregnancies. The prevailing view among researchers, however, is that alcohol's effects on development lie on a dose-dependent continuum and that lower levels of drinking, even "social" drinking, may also have some measurable effects on development.

The Seattle Pregnancy and Health Study has been examining the effects of a broad range of maternal drinking levels for several years in a longitudinal study. The research, involving a population sample of 500 women and their children, is designed to relate self-reported drinking levels during pregnancy to measurements of child development at birth, eight and 18 months, and at four to seven years of age.

Followup studies on the children have now been completed through age four, and several neurological and behavioral effects have been found in children whose mothers consumed alcohol either lightly, moderately, or fairly heavily during pregnancy. On several measures the effects are proportional to the level of alcohol consumption during pregnancy, and the data so far does not suggest a threshold level of drinking below which there is no effect on the unborn child.

Among the dose-dependent effects of prenatal alcohol exposure found in the children when they were newborns were impaired ability to "tune-out" and stop responding to a repeated extraneous stimulation, weaker sucking reflex, increased body tremors, and less vigorous body activity.

These findings support the hypothesis that the effects of prenatal alcohol exposure lie on a dose-dependent continuum. It should also be noted that this study measures self-reported average alcohol consumption levels and is not designed to take sporadic episodes of heavy drinking into account. A drinking binge occurring at a critical period of vulnerability during development could pose greater risks. Finally, although effects measured in a population may be small at lower drinking levels, there may well be subgroups in the population who are more susceptible than average to fetal alcohol effects at social drinking levels. There is no way to identify such subgroups at the present time. Until further research clarifies susceptibility factors, all women are well advised to avoid drinking during pregnancy.

9   FETAL ALCOHOL SYNDROME

A CRISIS FOR SOCIETY: THE POINT

E. Virginia Lapham

E. Virginia Lapham is Director of Social Work and Associate Professor in the Department of Pediatrics at Georgetown University. She is also Associate Director of the Department of Social Work at Georgetown University Hospital.

Points to Consider:

1. What experience with Fetal Alcohol Syndrome (FAS) does the author have?

2. Why is Fetal Alcohol Syndrome (FAS) a crisis for babies?

3. How is (FAE) or Fetal Alcohol Effects different from (FAS) Fetal Alcohol Syndrome?

4. Why is FAS a crisis for families and society?

Excerpted from testimony by E. Virginia Lapham before the Subcommittee on Children, Family, Drugs and Alcoholism of the Senate Committee on Labor and Human Resources, May 12, 1987.

***Fetal Alcohol Syndrome is one of the three leading
causes of mental retardation and the only one that is
entirely preventable.***

Each year in the United States, an estimated 40,000 babies
are born with physical and mental birth defects that are the
direct result of maternal ingestion of alcohol during pregnancy.
Alcohol during pregnancy is a crisis for the unborn. The birth of
a child with alcohol-related birth defects is also a crisis for
families and for society.

As part of my work at Georgetown University Child
Development Center, I have both direct involvement and
supervisory responsibilities for social work with high risk
pregnant women, with interdisciplinary assessments of infants,
children and youth who have a wide variety of chronic illnesses
and disabilities including alcohol-related birth defects.
Additionally, I spend one day each week in a treatment program
for severely mentally retarded and multihandicapped adults who
are being deinstitutionalized. Some of these adults also
evidence disabilities related to fetal alcohol syndrome. . .

Alcohol: Crisis for the Unborn

In 1973, Fetal Alcohol Syndrome (FAS) was officially identified
and labeled by Kenneth Jones and David Smith at the University
of Washington in Seattle. FAS is categorized by a cluster of
birth defects that include the following:

- growth retardation
- abnormalities of the face and head
- central nervous system dysfunction
- malformation of other organs or systems

Fetal Alcohol Syndrome is one of the three leading causes of
mental retardation and the only one that is entirely preventable.
The estimated incidence of FAS in the United States is
approximately one in 750 live births or 4,800 babies each year.

Infants who display less than four of the characteristics listed
are considered to have Fetal Alcohol Effects (FAE). The less
severe effects are believed to be associated with smaller
amounts of alcohol consumption during pregnancy and/or
different sensitivities of the fetus to the amount of alcohol that
crosses the placental barrier. For some infants, one drink may
be harmful, whereas in other cases, large amounts of alcohol
seem to have little effect. The effects also vary with the stage of
fetal development although no period of pregnancy is
considered safe and without risk. An estimated 36,000
newborns may be affected by FAE each year.

Questions are also being raised by child development

researchers about the relationship between fetal alcohol and the large number of children who are identified at school age as having attentional deficit disorders, learning disabilities, behavioral disturbances, and other symptoms often related to neurological dysfunction. If this relationship is found to be accurate, the actual numbers of children affected by alcohol in utero may eventually be found to be several times the current estimates, perhaps as high as one in 100 live births. A large number of spontaneous miscarriages are also considered to be due to alcohol use.

Life Long Impairments

Fetal Alcohol Syndrome and Fetal Alcohol Effects are life long impairments for the children affected. Early identification and intervention can help to improve the overall functioning level of the child by maximizing strengths and preventing social and emotional problems. Many of the affected children, perhaps most of the affected children, however, are not receiving needed services at an early age.

Fetal Alcohol: Crisis for Families

Babies with alcohol-related birth defects are born to parents with a wide range of family characteristics across all income and educational levels, racial and ethnic groups, age of parents, number of other children, and geographic locations. The one thing they have in common is that the mother used alcohol during part or all of her pregnancy.

Some babies are born to families in which the mother's drinking is done without knowledge of the consequences. In one case, the woman's physician even encouraged her to relax with a glass or two of wine with dinner each evening and she had not been able to stop with that amount. This mother may be one of those individuals with a genetic predisposition to alcoholism in which the individual has no control over the

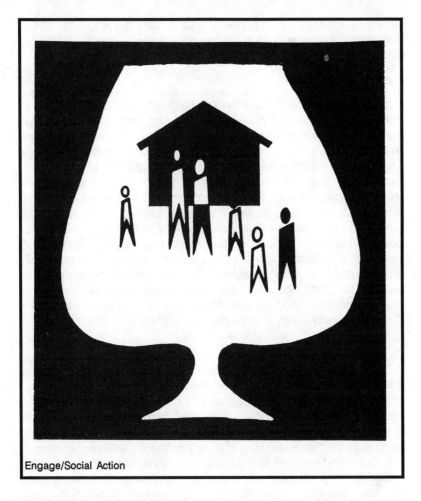

drinking from the first taste.

In another case of a mother with two older normal children whose husband had taken a job that required extensive periods of time away from home, the mother did binge drinking to try and cope with her loneliness. In this case, the baby was diagnosed with FAS soon after birth and the father learned for the first time about his wife's drinking. He was consumed with guilt for leaving his wife alone during the pregnancy while the mother also felt guilty about not being able to control her drinking.

With increased alcohol use among adolescents, some severely affected babies are born to teen mothers. Often these young women from high income as well as low income families have poor nutrition during pregnancy. When these adolescent mothers are also single and have inadequate or late prenatal care, the problems for the fetus may be additive and the outcome even worse. For these adolescent mothers and other mothers with additional life stress problems and few social supports, the care of a baby with birth defects is highly problematic.

Caring for Babies

Babies born with Fetal Alcohol Syndrome are often difficult to care for. Because of their small size and birth anomolies, they frequently remain in intensive care nurseries for weeks and even months. Their impaired nervous systems make them irritable, and they are not easily soothed by being held and cuddled. Sometimes they even have an aversion to touch and withdraw from the affection of their caretakers. The babies are often difficult to feed and may experience failure to thrive. Their development is slow, eye contact is poor, there are fewer smiles and the babies provide less satisfaction in parenting than normal babies. It is difficult for any parent to provide an optimal family environment for these babies. For parents who expected to have a laughing, cooing baby who would show unconditional love for them, the disappointment and difficulties of caring for the infants puts them at high risk for neglect and abuse.

Caring for Mothers

The mothers of babies born with FAS may also need special attention. Women who drink alcohol do so for a variety of reasons and with varying degrees of control. Women who drink primarily to facilitate socialization and can stop drinking at any time are probably the most amenable to an educational approach to cease drinking during pregnancy. Some women in this category may be risk takers and drink periodically anyhow believing they will beat the odds, and some do. They may even cite the data that show that "only 40 percent" of heavy drinkers have FAS children so how can an occasional drink be harmful? . .

Women who are physically dependent on alcohol and drink five or more drinks daily are at highest risk for having babies with the full blown Fetal Alcohol Syndrome and the least likely to abstain from drinking on their own. These are also the women who often get poor prenatal care and may have poor nutrition which adds to their problems and the problems of their unborn children. Intensive day treatment programs or even inpatient treatment may be indicated for pregnant women who are alcoholic, but denial is common and compliance rare. While the media have cited a few instances of pregnant alcoholic and/or drug abusing women being forced into treatment, this raises other kinds of ethical and legal questions of rights and responsibilities.

Welfare System

The children of alcoholic women often end up in the child welfare system either voluntarily because the parents are unable to provide care, or involuntarily because of neglect or abuse. Sometimes this occurs even before the baby is discharged from the hospital. Parents who fail to visit their babies in the intensive care nursery or who visit while under the influence of drugs or alcohol are reported to protective services for a home assessment before the hospital will discharge the baby. If the home is found unsafe, the baby may be turned over to a foster care agency and eventually released for adoption.

Adoptive and foster families are another category of families who often need help in understanding and providing optimal care for babies with alcohol-related birth defects who already have one strike against them. In one case of a single adoptive parent: the mother knew her four year old daughter had Fetal Alcohol Syndrome but as it turned out she didn't know what FAS implied for her daughter's development. She placed the child in a highly competitive private school with class sizes of 30 with one teacher. Each day the mother received reports from the school of her child's "bad behavior." The self-esteem of the child and the mother-child relationship were at risk when this mother joined a parent support group and received help from the other parents and from the group leader. . .

Fetal Alcohol Effects: Crisis for Society

The human and economic costs of having more than 40,000 infants born each year with Fetal Alcohol Syndrome and Fetal Alcohol Effects can only be surmised. The initial costs of 24 hour care in intensive care nurseries, medical and rehabilitative follow-up, special education, therapies, vocational or sheltered workshop training, adult underemployment or unemployment, residential care or supervision, and income assistance are all financial considerations to society. When children end up in the foster care or other branches of the child welfare system, the costs to society further increase.

One analysis of costs associated with FAS produced the following 1980 estimates: $14.9 million for health treatment of babies born with FAS; $670 million in total treatment costs for the 68,000 FAS children under the age of 18; $760 million in treatment costs for 160,000 FAS adults; and $510.5 million in indirect productivity losses. . .

Summary

1. An estimated 40,000 babies are born each year in the U.S. with alcohol-related birth defects. The actual figures may be higher.

2. Alcohol is a crisis for the unborn and subsequently for

families and for society.

3. Alcohol-related birth defects affect all segments of society.

4. The effects to the children are life long.

5. The resulting mental retardation and other nervous system dysfunctions are entirely preventable from a physiological perspective.

6. More information is needed about successful ways to help women refrain from alcohol during pregnancy.

7. Family stresses, including those related to alcohol abuse, may lead to abuse and neglect and further add to the problems of the affected children.

8. The U.S. public is not sufficiently aware of the risks of alcohol during pregnancy.

9. The human and economic costs of alcohol-related birth defects are staggering to consider and need to be calculated in more precise dollar figures.

10. Alcohol and drug treatment counselors and professionals who diagnose and treat children with alcohol-related birth defects have little knowledge and understanding of each other's expertise and interventions.

11. Research in prevention and treatment of alcohol-related birth defects is inadequate.

MISDIRECTED CRUSADE: THE COUNTERPOINT

Stanton Peele

Stanton Peele is a psychologist and health researcher at Mathematical Policy Research Institute, Princeton University. He is the author of Diseasing of America: Addiction Treatment Out of Control.

Points to Consider:

1. How does the author describe the book by Michael Dorris called *The Broken Cord?*

2. Describe the reasons for the author's belief that the dangers of fetal alcohol syndrome (FAS) and fetal alcohol effecfts (FAE) have been greatly exaggerated.

3. Who is Ralph Hingson and what did his study show?

4. Why has the crusade against drinking during pregnancy been misdirected?

5. Is any level of drinking safe during pregnancy?

The women most likely to give birth to damaged babies are not affected by messages tailored to the middle class.

A growing number of pregnant women in the United States avoid alcohol as if it were thalidomide. The pronouncements of government officials, journalists, and other professional alarmists have convinced them that drinking any amount of alcohol during pregnancy endangers the fetus. This new conventional wisdom is embodied in the federal warning that now appears on every bottle of wine, beer, and liquor manufactured for sale in this country: "According to the Surgeon General, women should not drink alcoholic beverages during pregnancy because of the risk of birth defects."

Campaigns

The horrible effects of fetal alcohol syndrome—which include mental retardation, cardiac defects, and facial deformities—were publicized throughout the 1980s. More recently, *The Broken Cord,* Michael Dorris's account of his experiences in raising an adopted Native American child suffering from FAS, has renewed the storm of anxiety about alcohol consumption during pregnancy. Dorris's book warns people that the danger of drinking by pregnant women has been vastly underestimated. The news media has been eager to amplify that view.

The success of the campaign against drinking during pregnancy demonstrates that any attacks on alcohol, no matter how far-fetched, misleading, or counter-productive, are nowadays immune from criticism. By blurring important distinctions, reports on FAS have generated needless worry among occasional or moderate drinkers while distracting attention from the real problems of prenatal care.

Research

People have long recognized that heavy alcohol consumption is a risky behavior for pregnant women. But U.S. researchers first used the term fetal alcohol syndrome in the early 1970s to describe severe abnormalities in the newborn children of alcoholic mothers, including brain damage and readily observable physical deformities.

Such children are quite rare, however, even among heavy drinkers. In their 1984 book *Alcohol and the Fetus,* based on a comprehensive survey of the research, Dr. Henry Rosett and Lyn Weiner of Boston University reported that studies find FAS occurs in only 2 percent to 10 percent of children born to alcohol abusers. Furthermore, they reported that in every one of the 400 FAS cases described in the scientific literature, the mother "was a chronic alcoholic who drank heavily during pregnancy."

The infrequency of FAS has prompted researchers to expand their focus beyond the severe birth defects sometimes caused by heavy drinking. Hence "fetal alcohol effect," which refers to more subtle impairment that might ordinarily escape attention. Closely tied to the rather vague notion of fetal alcohol effect is the suggestion that light or moderate drinking might also be dangerous. Warnings about FAS, fetal alcohol effect, and the alleged risks of any drinking during pregnancy get tossed together in the news media.

A February article by Dr. Elisabeth Rosenthal in *The New York Times Magazine*, "When a Pregnant Woman Drinks," begins with a horrific tale of an FAS victim. In this case, not only did the eight-year-old girl have FAS, but so did her siblings and her mother. Immediately following this extreme example, the article describes how Dr. Claire Coles, as FAS expert, has begun to "see the survivors of drinking pregnancies everywhere." For example, upon visiting a reform school, Coles observed, "My God, half these kids look alcohol-affected."

False Impressions

The bait-and-switch juxtaposition of Coles's observation with the severe FAS case creates the false impression that such alcohol-related birth defects are common. Alcohol-affected, the term used by Coles, is generally applied to infants who have problems that fall short of FAS, such as irritability, attention deficits, hyperactivity, or developmental delays. The condition cannot be discerned simply by looking at a child. But for those who see fetal alcohol effect "everywhere," even criminal behavior may be the result of a mother's drinking. (Attorneys representing condemned California murderer Robert Alton Harris offered such an argument.)

Increasingly, problems such as delinquency and learning

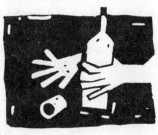

disabilities are being attributed to maternal drinking. Combined with warnings about moderate alcohol consumption, this tendency is likely to cause irrational guilt among many parents. The mother of a child who gets into trouble or has difficulty in school will start to wonder if this has anything to do with the wine she occasionally drank during her pregnancy.

Weiner, co-author of *Alcohol and the Fetus*, has described the anxiety caused by exaggeration of the danger from drinking during pregnancy: "Women are worrying about wine vinegar in their salad dressing and getting hysterical about the risk of eating rum cake, and they think they need an abortion after they hear the scare stories."

What grounds, if any, are there for such alarm? Rosenthal's article is accompanied by a subhead that warns, "New Studies Show that Even Moderate Consumption Can Be Harmful to the Unborn Child." But the article cites only one study to support this claim: In 1988, a University of Pittsburgh researcher found "minor anomalies" in children of mothers who consumed less than one drink a day during pregnancy.

Rosenthal has latched onto one highly unusual finding in a sea of contradictory evidence, ignoring a host of studies that have found no effect from consumption of two drinks a day or less. In 1984, Rosett and Weiner concluded, "the recommendation that all women should abstain from drinking during pregnancy is not based on scientific evidence." The overwhelming majority of studies since then have also failed to find evidence that moderate drinking harms the fetus. In fact, Dr. Jack Mendelson, a distinguished alcohol researcher at Harvard Medical School, has declared, "It is possible that some doses of alcohol, low or moderate, may improve the probability for healthy pregnancies and healthy offspring."

Lack of Evidence

Given the rush to condemn any drinking during pregnancy despite the lack of research evidence to support such a policy, you might guess that fetal alcohol effect, if not FAS itself, is a widespread phenomenon. But the Centers for Disease Control estimate that 8,000 "alcohol-damaged babies" are born each year, which works out to a rate of 2.7 for every 1,000 live births (0.27 percent).

Yet *New York Times* health columnist Jane Brody offered a much higher figure in 1986, when she announced, "An estimated 50,000 babies born last year suffered from prenatal alcohol exposure." (Brody, by the way, does not think it's enough merely to abstain from alcohol during pregnancy: "Even drinking before pregnancy [as little as one drink a day] may have a negative result," she reported.)

Rosenthal does not offer her own estimate, but she says the CDC figure seems low, apparently because "on some Indian reservations, 25 percent of all children are reportedly afflicted." But as she later notes, "The CDC data show that the syndrome is 30 times more commonly reported in Native Americans than it is in whites, and six times more common in blacks." These figures indicate that alcohol-related damage among babies of white, middle-class women is actually less common than 2.7 cases per 1,000, since all groups are averaged together in producing the overall rate.

Middle-Class Women

Indeed, it's not clear what the middle-class women who read the Times can learn from the experience of grossly dysfunctional families such as the one described at the beginning of Rosenthal's article or from reports about Native American children such as the mentally retarded in *The Broken Cord*. For one thing, styles of drinking vary widely across racial and socioeconomic groups.

White, middle-class women are more likely to drink than black women (and low-income women generally), but they tend to drink moderately. Black women are more likely to abstain, but those who don't are more likely to drink heavily. The fact that FAS rates are much higher among low-income minorities therefore contradicts the hypothesis that moderate drinking during pregnancy is damaging and that higher rates of abstinence would reduce FAS.

And a 1982 study by Boston University researcher Ralph Hingson suggests that other factors in the lives of poor, ghetto-dwelling women contribute to birth defects that have been ascribed solely to alcohol. After studying a sample of 1,700 women in Boston City Hospital, Hingson concluded that "neither level of drinking prior to pregnancy nor during pregnancy was significantly related to infant growth measures, congenital abnormality, or [other] features compatible with fetal alcohol syndrome."

Misdirected Crusade

Rather, a combination of factors—including smoking, malnutrition, and poor health care—seems to be responsible for low birth weight and other problems often attributed to drinking. "The results underline the difficulty in isolating and proclaiming single factors as the cause of abnormal fetal development," Hingson and his colleagues wrote.

So the crusade against drinking during pregnancy is misdirected in several ways. It focuses on moderate rather than heavy drinking, on middle-class rather than low-income mothers, and on alcohol consumption rather than the set of behaviors that increases the risk of birth defects. The women most likely to give birth to damaged babies—the ones who abuse alcohol and drugs, smoke, and neglect their health—are not affected by messages tailored to the middle class.

The error in strategy is especially troubling given the nation's relatively poor performance in prenatal care. The number of birth defects in the United States has doubled in the last 25 years. While the U.S. neonatal death rate dropped in the 1980s, it still compares unfavorably with those of European nations, Japan, Australia, Singapore, Bermuda, and even Guam. Shrill warnings about low levels of drinking during pregnancy may make health experts feel virtuous, but they won't improve those figures one bit. Developing comprehensive community programs for high-risk mothers would help, but this requires more than Sunday-supplement alarmism.

What Is Editorial Bias?

This activity may be used as an individualized study guide for students in libraries and resource centers or as a discussion catalyst in small group and classroom discussions.

The capacity to recognize an author's point of view is an essential reading skill. The skill to read with insight and understanding involves the ability to detect different kinds of opinions or bias. Sex bias, ethnocentric bias, political bias and religious bias are five basic kinds of opinions expressed in editorials and all literature that attempts to persuade. They are briefly defined in the glossary below.

Glossary of Terms for Reading Skills

SEX BIAS — the expression of dislike for and/or feeling of superiority over the opposite sex or a particular sexual minority

RACE BIAS — The expression of dislike for and/or feeling of superiority over a racial group

ETHNOCENTRIC BIAS — The expression of a belief that one's own group, race, religion, culture or nation is superior. Ethnocentric persons judge others by their own standards and values.

POLITICAL BIAS — the expression of political opinions and attitudes about domestic or foreign affairs

RELIGIOUS BIAS — the expression of a religious belief or attitude

Guidelines

1. From the readings in Chapter Three, locate five sentences that provide examples of editorial opinion or bias.

2. Write down each of the above sentences and determine what kind of bias each sentence represents. Is it *sex bias, race bias, ethnocentric bias, political bias or religious bias?*

3. Make up a one sentence statement that would be an example of each of the following: *sex bias, race bias, ethnocentric bias, political bias and religious bias.*

4. See if you can locate five sentences that are factual statements from the readings in Chapter Three.

CHAPTER 4

FETAL NEGLECT AND SOCIAL RESPONSE

11 FETAL NEGLECT AND SOCIAL RESPONSE

MORE SOCIAL PROGRAMS NEEDED TO PREVENT PERINATAL DRUG ABUSE

Wendy Chavkin

Wendy Chavkin, M.D. is a Rockefeller Fellow at the Sergiersky Center, Columbia University School of Public Health.

Points to Consider:

1. Explain what the data say about pregnant women using illicit drugs.

2. How has society responded to the problem of perinatal drug abuse?

3. Under what circumstances has criminal prosecution been used?

4. What are the treatment options for drug abusive pregnant women?

Wendy Chavkin in testimony before the House Select Committee on Children, Youth and Families, April 27, 1989.

It is widespread practice in New York City to screen neonatal urine for the presence of illicit drugs when maternal substance use is suspected.

Although baseline data are sparse, all the evidence suggests that there has indeed been a sizeable increase in the numbers of women using illicit drugs (primarily crack) during pregnancy.

In New York City, for example, the number of birth certificates indicating maternal substance use has tripled from 730 in 1981 (6.7/100 livebirths) to 2586 f(20.3/1000 livebirths) in 1987.

Criminal Prosecution

There have been three major categories of societal response to this problem. The one that has attracted the most media attention, but is the rarest, has been the criminal prosecution of new mothers for their use of illicit drugs during pregnancy. As fetal personhood is not legally recognized, these have involved various legal approaches. In California, in the Reyes case of 1977 and the widely publicized Stewart case of 1986, attempts were made to prosecute two women on grounds of criminal child abuse. Since the fetus is not recognized as a child, the statutes were deemed inapplicable and the cases dismissed. Subsequently the local prosecutor in northern California's Butte County has announced his intention of using a positive newborn toxicology screen in the baby as evidence of maternal illicit drug use, a prosecutable offense. Currently in Florida, Toni Suzette Hudson is facing charges of "transferring an illicit drug from one person to another", because of her prenatal crack use for which she faces a possible 30-year sentence if convicted. In another twist, last year in Washington D.C., Brenda Vaughn was convicted of forging a check to support her drug habit. As she was a first-time offender, she would normally have been put on probation. However, when the judge learned she was pregnant, he decided to incarcerate her for the duration of the pregnancy, stating he "would be darned if he'd have a baby born addicted."

The move toward criminal prosecution reflects, I believe, deep-seated ambivalence about whether addiction constitutes willful criminal behavior or a medical illness, despite two Supreme Court decisions (in 1925 in the Linden case and again in 1962 in Robinson vs. California) that addiction was an illness. The move also reflects a tendency, which I believe has its roots in the anti-abortion movement, to view pregnant woman and fetus as separate with competing, even antagonistic interests. Whereas previously pregnant women with alcohol or drug addiction problems were considered in need of help, now some perceive them as willful wrongdoers toward the fetus.

Child Neglect

The second major category of response has been invocation of the child neglect apparatus. Some states — New York is one — consider parental habitual drug use as prima facie evidence of child neglect.

It is widespread practice in New York City to screen neonatal urine for the presence of illicit drugs when maternal substance use is suspected. Criteria for suspicion vary and are rarely articulated in protocols. A positive toxicology screen is interpreted as evidence of maternal repeated illicit substance use, and therefore prima facie evidence of neglect, and triggers a mandatory report to Special Services for Children (SSC). SSC then conducts an investigation, and if it deems the woman to be a neglectful parent, the agency files charges in Family Court, and places the child in foster care. Because of the increasing number of such cases and the shortage of foster homes, these investigations are often prolonged, and in the interim the babies board in hospitals or congregate in care facilities (institutional care for 6-24 babies, run by the city). In 1987 at the first peak of the boarder baby crisis in New York City, maternal substance use was the primary reason for boarder baby status, accounting for 40% of 300 plus cases. Approximately one-third of these drug exposed infants were ultimately discharged to the biological family after boarding in hospitals an average of 50-60 days. A recent report by the New York City Comptroller indicated that maternal drug use (48%) and inadequate housing (49%) were the two primary reasons for boarder status, and that there are approximately 300 children under two years of age boarding in a hospital on any given day.

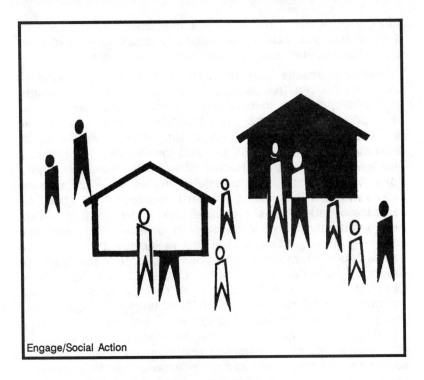

Engage/Social Action

Drug Treatment and Prenatal Care

The third category of societal response is to offer drug treatment and prenatal care for addicted women. Various federal agencies and the Surgeon General have extensively documented this nation's failure to provide prenatal care for all who need it. Unfortunately the situation regarding drug treatment for pregnant women is even worse. I recently concluded a survey of 78 drug treatment programs in New York City (95% of the total). Fifty-four percent refused to treat pregnant women; 67% refused to treat pregnant women on Medicaid, and 87% had no services available to pregnant women on Medicaid addicted to crack. Less than half of those programs that did accept pregnant women (44%) provided or arranged for prenatal care; only two programs made provisions for clients' children. Yet lack of child care is a major obstacle to participation in drug treatment for many women, as the National Institute for Drug Abuse (NIDA) documented a decade ago.

Lack of Treatment Options

This lack of treatment options for pregnant women reflects a legacy of discrimination against women addicts by drug treatment programs, which was reported by the National Institute of Drug Abuse a decade ago. It also reflects medical uncertainty over the optimal medical management of addiction during pregnancy. Other treatment modalities for the treatment of crack addiction include psychotherapy, acupuncture and other medications (certain antidepressants and anticonvulsants). . .

Promising results have been reported from the handful of programs around the country. . .Several of these programs emphasize parenting training and consider parent education to be a critical component. The Perinatal Addiction Center at Northwestern Hospital in Chicago, the Family Care Center at Jefferson Hospital in Philadelphia and the Program for Pregnant Addicts and Addicted Mothers at Metropolitan Hospital in New York City are three such successful examples. The Acupuncture Drug Treatment Program at Lincoln Hospital in New York City has recently added on-site prenatal care and pregnancy-related health education and is developing on-site child care and parenting classes. Others urge that residential drug treatment be available for mothers with young children. The Mabond Program Family Center, part of the Odyssey House Therapeutic Community on Wards Island in New York provides residential treatment for 30 women with children under the age of five years. The women can pursue high school equivalency diplomas, job training and placement because of the on-site provision of day care. Parenting education and early childhood stimulation are considered key components of the program.

The society must choose whether to allocate resources to therapy or to sanction. Even the criminal and child neglect models presuppose the availability of therapy, as an addict cannot conform her behavior to the requirements of the law otherwise.

12 FETAL NEGLECT AND SOCIAL RESPONSE

STRICT LAWS NEEDED TO PROTECT THE UNBORN

Esther D. March

Esther March is the Discharge Planner and Parent Educator in the Neonatal Intensive Care Unit at Broward General Medical Center in Fort Lauderdale, Florida.

Points to Consider:

1. What experience did the author have with premature and sick newborns?

2. Explain the problems of cocaine-addicted parents with newborn infants.

3. Why are babies sometimes discharged from hospitals to drug-addicted mothers?

4. What solutions are suggested for this problem?

Esther D. March in testimony before the House Select Committee on Narcotics Abuse and Control, October 16, 1987.

Many babies are still being discharged to mothers who have not received any drug treatment.

I have worked in the Neonatal Intensive Care Unit for many years. As the Discharge Planner and Parent Educator, I function as a liaison between the community and hospital systems preparing for the infants' discharge. Many of these infants require special medical care at home and their parent(s) must learn additional caretaking skills in order for the infant to thrive. My job is to prepare parents to care for these infants' special needs at home and to link them with a multitude of supportive community agencies for follow-up care.

With the birth of a premature or sick newborn, there is a series of psycho-social problems or crises that the parents must face. These problems or crises can be, and many times are, worked out by the parents before the infant is discharged. What concerns me the most is the unresolved psycho-social problems that many of the neonatal parents are faced with because of their cocaine addiction. They often have unstable housing, few resources and are functioning at such a low level that they cannot, or choose not to seek public assistance.

Caring for Infants

These parents' physical condition, lack of motivation, and lack of attachment to their infants, makes it very difficult to teach the many special skills that are needed for their infants' home care. In the Neonatal Unit, many cocaine-addicted parents have displayed their inability to care for their infants because of their rapid mood changes, their lack of coordination, and the fact that they often cannot recall information that is vital to the infant's survival.

I am aware that a referral system was implemented last year to address the problems dealing with pregnant women and cocaine abuse; however, this program has not met the community needs. Many babies are still being discharged to mothers who have not received any drug treatment either because they have refused to acknowledge their problem, or because of a lack of available in-patient beds for the indigent population.

Case Example One:

I recall a situation that happened two weeks ago when a mother gave birth to a premature baby boy. The baby remained in the hospital for seven days. Because of the mother's drug history and the baby's positive urine test for cocaine, a Public Health referral was made. A home investigation was performed, and the report revealed open drug activity going on between the baby's mother and three men. Two days later a second home

TESTING PREGNANT WOMEN

For the first time, doctors in Minnesota must test pregnant women for drug use, even without the patient's consent, if there's reason to suspect even casual drug use. Test results that indicate drug use then must be reported to local child-welfare agencies for follow-up.

Maura Lerner, Star Tribune *of Minneapolis, January 15, 1990*

investigation was performed which revealed no open drug activity at that time. The home investigation was deemed satisfactory for the infant's discharge. This mother came to the hospital for the infant's discharge without any baby supplies or equipment, and alcohol was noted on her breath. The child was released to the custody of his mother with only Public Health follow-up.

Case Example Two:

Another case example is a single mother who gave birth to a severely premature male infant who remained in the hospital for three months. The child was ventilated and required multiple procedures which required parental consent. Because of the mother's unstable housing situation, it was nearly impossible to locate her in a timely manner for ongoing consultation regarding her infant's progress and medical treatment. Throughout this baby's three month hospitalization, the mother visited three times. She got minimally involved in his care despite encouragement and support for this by nursing staff. Upon discharge, this infant required medication and an apnea home monitor. I made several appointments for teaching of CPR and home monitor training which the mother did not keep. After being threatened with an abandonment referral, the mother showed up four days after the scheduled discharge date to take her baby home. This mother marginally completed required training for her infant's care, but was noted to fall asleep while feeding him. Despite my feeling of uneasiness in releasing this child to his mother, the system as it now exists, left me no recourse but to discharge this child home.

I feel that these two babies and all other babies with similar circumstances should be protected by the legal system until the parents receives treatment for their drug addiction. These infants are at very high risk for abuse and neglect, and in many cases, because of the powerful addiction, the driving force in the parents' life is the substance that they are addicted to, and the parents' drug needs will be given priority over the needs of their infants. Treatment should be court ordered when a mother

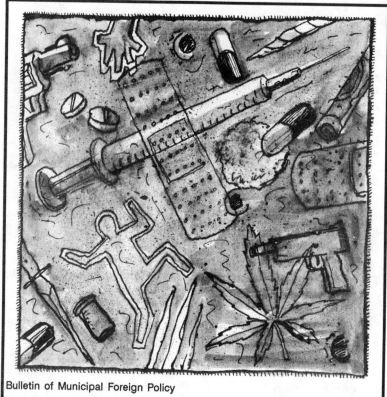

Bulletin of Municipal Foreign Policy

refuses to acknowledge her problem. Until treatment is completed, the children should be placed in legal custody of a significant other or in an alternative care situation. This will ensure the protection of the children and provide support for the persons who are often put in the position of primary caretaker because of the mother's dysfunction. In many cases, these significant others lack legal support to safeguard the child and make important decisions related to the child's needs because they are not considered legal guardians.

Summary

The drug referral system has been an asset in identifying many high risk drug cases, but there is a tremendous need for legislation of resources to help treat the parent(s) with the addiction and to place the infant in a safe environment during the parent(s)' treatment process. Within the present legal system, only those drug addicted infants who are abandoned may be referred to protective services from the hospital setting. I believe the future of our country depends upon the healthy, physical and emotional development of our children.

13   FETAL NEGLECT AND SOCIAL PROBLEMS

BIRTH CONTROL AND PREVENTION IS THE ANSWER

Esther Wattenberg

Esther Wattenberg is a professor in the School of Social Work and associate for the Center for Urban and Regional Affairs at the University of Minnesota.

Points to Consider:

1. How is the power of the state to rescue children from harm described?

2. What is eugenics and why can it not be used to deal with the problem of drug addicted babies?

3. Identify strategies that have failed to prevent prenatal drug abuse.

4. Describe the strategies that can help to prevent the birth of babies damaged by drug addicted pregnant women.

Esther Wattenberg, "Prevention Should Be the First Step," *Star Tribune,* August 13, 1989. Reprinted with permission of *Star Tribune.*

How can we reduce the problem of unwanted children, the source of a significant number of abuse and neglect cases?

With each exposé of a child dying from neglect, injured by a brutal physical attack, condemned to a deformed life from being poisoned in the womb by a drug- or alcohol-addicted mother, the public erupts in anger and frustration with a system that doesn't work.

Power of the State

Missing from the dissection of child abuse cases is a stubborn truth: The power of the state to rescue children from harm is severely limited. Errors are inherent in a complicated system designed to protect children.

Sorting out the degree of danger, weighing the evidence of abuse and neglect and judging the capacity of a family to change requires the wisdom of Solomon. Furthermore, decisions are enmeshed in the contradiction of a society that wants to guarantee the privacy of a family and its right to rear children within its own values, and that, at the same time, wants to protect children from harm.

Even social workers, police, psychiatrists, mental health workers, nurses and doctors do not always agree on how to deal with vulnerable children in life-threatening environments. Fools rush in. Angels fear to tread. Procedures are fallible. The system makes mistakes.

And yet reports, studies and newspaper articles such as the *Star Tribune's* "Fatal Neglect" are churned out as if tinkering with the system will protect children. The question is persistently raised: How can you make the system more responsive and effective?

Prevention

The more important question, and maybe the more difficult one, is rarely raised: How can we prevent child abuse? Really prevent—before harm occurs.

At first glance, it would seem easy to unify the community around a prevention plan. From bare-bone statistics, we know that the life prospects of 20 percent of children in any given year are grim. Isn't preventing abuse a worthy and major social challenge? Of course. But how?

Consider primary prevention: blocking high-risk men and women from having children.

We can identify the perpetrators of the worst child abuse. They are men and women who have a lethal combination of characteristics: violent, given to uncontrollable rages, immature, cruel in a primitive sense and perhaps mentally ill or mentally deficient. The key is their incapacity to love a child in a nurturing way.

Eugenics

We could all agree that this particular breed should never become parents. How to do that? Sterilization on the basis of some calculated formula of "perpetrator risk"? States have, from time to time, attempted to eradicate the "undesirables".

Even so notable a liberal judge as Justice Oliver Wendell Holmes was persuaded that the state could justify sterilization of incompetents. "...It is better for all the world, if instead of waiting to execute degenerate offspring for crime, or to let them starve for their imbecility, society can prevent those who are manifestly unfit from continuing their kind." (Buck vs. Bell, 1926)

Eugenic societies flourished before World War II, dedicated to improving the human race through genetic controls. The movement was brought to a halt with the unfolding horrors of the Nazis' dedication to purifying the Aryan race. The lesson of how a nation goes berserk in its zeal to purify itself is indelible. We should not revive eugenic arguments.

The inescapable truth is that we have no acceptable way of forcing those who should never be parents from not becoming parents. The preemptive strike is out.

Strategies

Well, then, how can we reduce the problem of unwanted children, the source of a significant number of abuse and neglect cases? Can we prevent conception when it is desperately unwelcome, as with school-age children and parents under intolerable stress? Can we make it possible for pregnancies to be terminated with the discovery of a badly deformed fetus? These are the conditions that yield a profile of

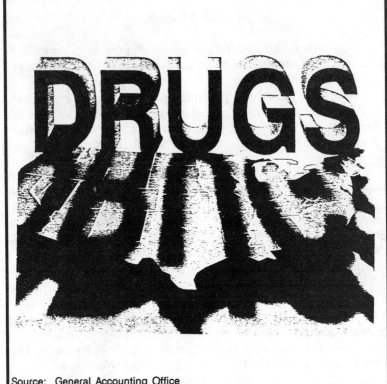

Source: General Accounting Office

risk for child abuse.

We know what to do: open access to contraception, school-based clinics, sex education and, yes, an affirmation of Roe vs. Wade abortion rights with Medicaid funding restored for poor women. While the community is deeply divided on these issues, we should face the real meaning of child abuse prevention: discouraging the repugnant pregnancy and the hateful birth of a rejected child.

A forceful argument could be made for adoption. But few women are willing to endure a nine month pregnancy and then give up the child. Less than five percent do so now, and the number is dwindling. If there are fresh strategies to encourage adoption, they merit support. But there are none on the horizon.

Education

The child abuse phenomenon has, at last, caught the attention of the public. We should not squander the moment. The community should be educated to understand that treating abusive families is a long, costly struggle with uncertain outcomes. But spare us the homilies about how to fix a problem which, in fact, is not amenable to easy answers.

Concentrate on prevention strategies. Should we fail at prevention, then a community that demands safety for children will have to dig deeply into its pockets to pay for it.

No illusions, please. Let us at least first try to prevent the tragedies of unwanted children.

14   FETAL NEGLECT AND SOCIAL RESPONSE

MORE TREATMENT PROGRAMS ARE NEEDED

Lucia Meijer

Lucia Meijer is a Substance Abuse Coordinator with the AIDS Education and Training Center for the University of Washington's Department of Medicine.

Points to Consider:

1. How is the relationship between treatment for women and their economics status described?

2. Why are few treatment programs designed to meet the need of women?

3. What principles of human behavior must be better understood?

4. Explain the author's recommendations for improving perinatal drug abuse treatment programs.

Lucia Meijer in testimony before the House Select Committee on Children, Youth and Families, April 27, 1989.

There is increasing concern over the trend towards the "feminization of poverty".

Despite an apparent proliferation of chemical dependency treatment programs throughout the country, there is reason to believe that females experiencing cocaine and other drug addictions may not be able to access or benefit from existing treatment services.

Uniformity

Treatment services are not uniformly available or utilized. The 1987 National Drug and Alcoholism Treatment Unit Survey (NDATUS) collected information on 8,690 facilities with a total of 614,123 clients on a given date (10/30/87) and 2,264,111 unduplicated clients over a 12 month period. The data in this report suggest that there are significant variations in treatment utilization, and that these differences may reflect a lack of availability of treatment to certain populations. . .

Women and Poverty

Economic limitations on treatment availability may have a disproportionate impact on addicted women. There is increasing concern over the trend towards the "feminization of poverty". Studies of drug dependent women (Sutker, 1981) indicate high levels of unemployment in this population (from 81% to 96%). Of the women in federally funded treatment programs, most had not completed high school. Even after completing treatment, 72% continued to be unemployed and lacked necessary skills to get or keep a job. It has been argued that the female addict is likely to be even more socially and economically dysfunctional than her male counterpart because of cultural stigmas against female drug use that increase her isolation from family and other socioeconomic supports.

Many female addicts are responsible for one or more children, and this further limits their ability to access or utilize educational and vocational options. AIDS related studies reveal that of the IV drug users that were in relationships, the majority of women had partners who were also drug users while almost 80% of the male IV users had non-drug using partners. The female addict is less likely to be able to rely on a more stable partner for support, yet she is more likely to be responsible for the care of children. High pregnancy and birth rates have been documented among female drug users (Deren, 1985) due in part to a lack of use of birth control.

Needs of Women

Few treatment programs are designed to meet the needs of women drug users. Because the actual number of women

JUNKIE MOTHERS

About 5.5 million of the 9.5 million drug users are now women.

All states report shortages in services for women. . .

An estimated 1 million drug-exposed babies will be born between 1988 and 1991. Each could cost up to $100,000 in intensive medical care. That means, ultimately, taxpayers will pay billions of dollars for that care. Perhaps only then junkie mothers might begin to get the help they need.

Fern Schumer, USA Today, *January 9, 1990*

in treatment is small, and because female addicts are more likely to be in highly utilized drug programs, specialized services for the addicted woman have not been a priority in the treatment system. Perhaps even more importantly, many programs lack the flexibility and skills to develop relevant programming for women. Most treatment approaches are based on the characteristics and dynamics of addiction among male populations, and comparatively little has been done to define the unique nature of addiction in women. If addiction is, in fact, a complex interaction of biological, psychological, and social factors, then differences in gender should be a primary variable in how addiction is developed and sustained.

Many programs operate from a single model of addiction and recovery, although current research suggests strongly that different types of clients require different treatments. This does not necessarily require more programs, just more effective use of existing services. McLellan et al. (1986) found that within a single program, clients who were matched to specialized services according to a variety of individual characteristics did better than those who were not matched. This prospective study also found that client-treatment matching methods made it possible to identify clients suited to less expensive out-patient and/or shorter term programs resulting in a more cost efficient use of resources (*"Drug Abuse and Drug Abuse Research, The Second Triennial Report to Congress From The Secretary, Department of Health and Human Services"*). . .

Changing Behavior

The effectiveness of existing programs in addressing the needs of addicted women may be increased through a better understanding and application of some basic principles of human behavior.

For any change to occur, three conditions must be met:

1. **The person must accept that she has a need to change.** This is commonly approached through confrontive methods meant to "break down the client's denial.". Research suggests that this method can have a negative effect on people with low self-esteem. Low self-esteem is a characteristic often found in female addicts. A more effective approach teaches the woman to identify and personalize information about her problem behaviors and circumstances.

2. **The benefits of change must outweigh the losses.** However dysfunctional, most behaviors are connected to needs that are intensely felt. All too often concern for the female addict focuses on her role as a "vector" of harm to others, and not as an individual deserving of concern and compassion in her own right. The woman's needs for safety, relief from pain, affiliation with others, etc., are all integral to the process of addiction. Treatment cannot be effective if it does not address the needs that fuel the addiction by providing alternative and more functional ways for the woman to meet these needs. This means providing achievable options for change that balance needs and risks, rather than drastic "all or nothing" objectives.

3. **The skills and resources necessary for change must be accessible.** Recovery often requires that the woman change important relationships and familiar circumstances. This requires internal skills and external resources including cognitive training, self-esteem building, communications skills, medical care, parenting skills, vocational training, child care options, educational and economic opportunities, etc. Skills and resources should be appropriate to the ability of the client to use them. For example, job training can be futile in the absence of reading skills. . .

More Treatment Programs

Recommendations:

1. **Increase supports for comprehensive perinatal substance abuse treatment programs.** There are only four programs specifically for pregnant addicts in the country — one in San Francisco, one in Los Angeles, one in Chicago, and one in Philadelphia (Cohen, et al., *The Journal of Drug Issues,* Winter 1989). This does not begin to match the need for such programs in light of the current epidemic of cocaine-addicted mothers and infants, and the increasing number of babies born with HIV infection.

2. **Increase the ability of states to access treatment monies.** A recent article in the *New York Times* reports that $777 million in federal funds available to states for drug education and rehabilitation have not been used and are due to expire on September 30, 1989. The reasons given for failure of many states to apply for the money included "a lack of state

programs that the federal funds are intended to help and slow-moving state governments that are confused by the federal formulas for allocating and using the money". (*New York Times,* Monday, April 17, 1989). If possible reduce the complexity of the application procedures, and provide federal leadership to facilitate the use of these funds.

3. **Focus funding opportunities on programs that service clients in low socio-economic groups.** Programs that target drug using populations appear to have the highest proportion of women in treatment. These programs rely far more on government funding than their alcohol or combined treatment counterparts that receive substantial private third party payments.

15   FETAL NEGLECT AND SOCIAL RESPONSE

A COMPREHENSIVE NATIONAL ANTI-DRUG STRATEGY IS NEEDED

Charles B. Rangel

Charles B. Rangel is a congressman from New York. He is the Chairman of the House Select Committee on Narcotics Abuse and Control.

Points to Consider:

1. How does the author describe the problem of maternal drug abuse?

2. What specific problems do babies display?

3. Why are drug addicted mothers not to blame for their problems?

4. Explain the need for drug treatment programs.

Charles B. Rangel in testimony before the House Select Committee on Children, Youth And Families, April 27, 1989.

Many of these children will experience a variety of potential long term problems such as mental retardation, hyperactivity, and learning disabilities.

As Chairman of the Select Committee on Narcotics Abuse and Control, as a state legislator, and as a prosecutor, I have for almost three decades witnessed the devastation and destruction wreaked by drug abuse. Nothing, however, has made me feel more helpless than watching the tiny bodies of infants squirming and shaking because of the effects of drug abuse. Nothing has made me more angry and determined to end the strangle hold of drugs on our society. . .

In July, 1987, the Select Committee on Narcotics held a hearing at Harlem Hospital in New York on intravenous drug abuse and pediatric AIDS. In October of 1987 the Committee visited Broward County Medical Center in Florida where we held a hearing on cocaine-addicted infants.

The Findings Were Devastating:

—the number of children born affected by maternal drug abuse was increasing;

—the range of effects was expanding; and

—not only were drug treatment services inadequate, but pregnant women were at times denied services even when they were available.

The present level of drug abuse in our society gives reason for continued alarm. An estimated 30 million Americans have used cocaine. Five to six million use cocaine regularly. Heroin abuse continues at significant levels with approximately 600,000 heroin addicts. Regular marijuana users number 25 million and another 15 million Americans may use it occasionally.

Women and Drugs

These statistics reflect an increase in drug use among women. Most of these women are in their child-bearing years. New York City alone, in 1987, reported 2,588 births to mothers using illicit drugs.

Among the five to six million regular cocaine users, an estimated two million are women. Moreover, women in their child-bearing years constitute an ever growing proportion of cocaine users. It has been estimated that 10 percent of pregnant women have tried cocaine at least once during their pregnancy.

Approximately 31 percent of American women in their late teens and twenties indicated in a 1985 survey that they had used marijuana within the last year. LSD, PCP, and heroin are also being used by young women. All of these substances used during pregnancy have the potential to seriously affect prenatal health and development.

This increase in drug use by young women is clearly responsible for the growing number of infants we are seeing being born suffering from the effects of maternal drug use. The range of effects is frightening.

The Children

Many of these children are born suffering from withdrawal or withdrawal-like symptoms. Some experience heart attacks, strokes, and respiratory problems. Still others are born prematurely, are smaller and have lower birth weights—factors that influence their development. There is also mounting evidence that many of these children are more vulnerable to Sudden Infant Death Syndrome (SIDS) or crib death. Moreover, preliminary reports indicate that many of these children will experience a variety of potential long term problems such as mental retardation, hyperactivity, and learning disabilities. Perhaps the most tragic of all are the children born suffering not only from the direct effects of drug addiction, but also from AIDS transmitted as a result of parental drug abuse.

Information regarding the effects of specific drugs on fetal development is meager, although research in this area has increased dramatically in the past few years. From a policy perspective, however, whether it is cocaine, heroin, or marijuana; a combination of drug; or a drug-related lifestyle that causes a particular problem of the newborn, the bottom line is that we must stop the use of drugs particularly among women in their child-bearing years.

The Mothers

How do we do this? It would be easy to point a finger at the mothers of these children, but that will not solve our problem. These mothers are not responsible for the bumper crops of coca, opium and marijuana in drug producing countries. They are not to blame for the influx of drugs into this country, because our borders are, for all intents and purposes, a sieve. And, it is not their fault that we have not had, until recently, federal funds for drug education or prevention programs. It is not the mothers who have promoted slogans rather than policies as the primary weapon against drug abuse. Finally, it is not the mothers who determine the availability and accessibility of drug treatment and prenatal care.

To prevent any more infants from becoming victims of cocaine abuse, our first line of defense must be a comprehensive national anti-drug strategy. The Anti-Drug Abuse Acts of 1986 and 1988 took us a step toward that objective. They provided new policies and additional assistance in the areas of international narcotics control; interdiction; drug law enforcement; and drug abuse treatment, education, and prevention.

Treatment

Especially critical to the specific problem of drug abusing women and their infants is the need for additional drug treatment resources. The Anti-Drug Abuse Act of 1986 and 1988 expanded resources for drug abuse treatment services. For 1989, $806 million was appropriated for the Federal Alcohol, Drug Abuse, and Mental Health Block Grants. Another $75 million was appropriated to reduce treatment waiting lists.

The need for treatment services, however, still far exceeds the availability of services. The National Institute on Drug Abuse estimates that there are 6.5 million people using drugs in a way that seriously impairs their health and ability to function. Yet nationwide, at any one time, there are only 240,000 drug abusers in treatment.

Moreover, the specific treatment needs of pregnant women and women in their child-bearing years are not being adequately addressed. The National Association of State Alcohol and Drug Abuse Directors in its 1987 report specifically identified drug treatment services for women and youth as an area of unmet need. Clearly, not only are additional treatment resources needed, but they must reach the very vulnerable population—women in their child-bearing years. . .

Child-Bearing Years

Much more must be done. There are a number of efforts that should be undertaken, which specifically target women in their child-bearing years, pregnant women who abuse drugs, and infants of drug abusing mothers.

—First, for high risk women who are pregnant and those in their child-bearing years there is a need for:

- early identification and referral to drug abuse treatment;

- available and accessible drug abuse treatment;
- available and accessible prenatal care (many women still only see an emergency room doctor at delivery);
- drug abuse prevention/education outreach programs.

Perhaps the services provided by drug treatment centers will have to be expanded to include providing primary health care services, and specifically gynecological and obstetrics services if we are to reach the drug users with desperately needed health care services.

—*Second, for the mothers after the birth of the child there is a need for:*

- training to meet the special needs of the child;
- social support services to reduce the possibility of child abuse or neglect;
- continued drug treatment with follow-up supports.

—*Third, for the child there is a need for:*

- better health care before birth;
- adequate health care after birth
- special services to meet long term needs, e.g., learning disabilities and behavioral problems;
- foster care and adoption services.

—*Fourth, we must also reach out to the medical profession.* It is they who must ensure that doctors are aware of the symptoms of drug use; inform their patients of the dangers of drug abuse, especially pregnant women and women in their child-bearing years; and respond to the patients' drug problem as part of their health care.

In closing, let me say, there is much to be done and it must be done soon, for we are risking the loss of future generations by our inactivity. While I applaud the initiative and creativity of the witnesses today who will be describing programs already underway to respond to the needs of the children who have been afflicted from birth with the curse of drug abuse and addiction, I am also deeply distressed that such programs are needed. As a father and legislator, I had hoped that we would leave a better America to the next generation. I still have that hope, but we will have to do much to redeem our society for our children.

Recognizing Author's Point of View

This activity may be used as an individualized study guide for students in libraries and resource centers or as a discussion catalyst in small group and classroom discussions.

Many readers are unaware that written material usually expresses an opinion or bias. The capacity to recognize an author's point of view is an essential reading skill. The skill to read with insight and understanding involves the ability to detect different kinds of opinions or bias. Sex bias, race bias, ethnocentric bias, political bias and religious bias are five basic kinds of opinions expressed in editorials and all literature that attempts to persuade. They are briefly defined in the glossary below.

Five Kinds of Editorial Opinion or Bias

SEX BIAS—the expression of dislike for and/or feeling of superiority over the opposite sex or a particular sexual minority

RACE BIAS— the expression of dislike for and/or feeling of superiority over a racial group

ETHNOCENTRIC BIAS— the expression of a belief that one's own group, race, religion, culture or nation is superior. Ethnocentric persons judge others by their own standards and values.

POLITICAL BIAS—the expression of political opinions and attitudes about domestic or foreign affairs

RELIGIOUS BIAS—the expression of a religious belief or attitude

Guidelines

1. Locate three examples of political opinion or bias in the readings from Chapter Four.

2. Locate five sentences that provide examples of any kind of editorial opinion or bias from the readings in Chapter Four.

3. Write down each of the above sentences and determine what kind of bias each sentence represents. Is it **sex bias, race bias, ethnocentric bias, political bias or religious bias?**

4. Make up a one sentence statement that would be an example of each of the following: **sex bias, race bias, ethnocentric bias, political bias and religious bias.**

5. See if you can locate five sentences that are factual statements from the readings in Chapter Four.

Summarize the author's point of view in one sentence for each of the following:

Reading 11_____

Reading 12_____

Reading 13_____

Reading 14_____

Reading 15_____

CHAPTER 5

CRIME, PREGNANCY AND DRUGS

16 CRIME, PREGNANCY AND DRUGS

CRIMINAL PROSECUTION AND PREGNANT WOMEN: AN OVERVIEW

ABA Journal

Illegal drugs and abortion are probably the most emotionally charged social issues in the United States. So it comes as no surprise that tensions run high when legal cases raising questions of a woman's duty to her unborn child combine elements of both these social lightning rods.

Criminal Charges

In May, Melanie Green, 24, of Rockford, Ill., was charged with involuntary manslaughter and supplying drugs to a minor when her daughter, Bianca, died two days after birth. Cocaine was found in the baby's urine and mother's bloodstream. A grand jury later refused to bring an indictment against Green.

The criminal charges were the most serious to date involving a mother and her fetus.

Last year a Washington, D.C. superior court judge sent a pregnant woman, Brenda Vaughn, to jail on a second-degree theft conviction after she tested positive for cocaine use. (See "Pregnant? Go Directly to Jail," Nov.1, 1988, *ABA Journal*, page 20.)

In 1987, a Los Angeles municipal court judge dismissed charges against Pamela Rae Stewart, who was accused of contributing to her infant's death by taking drugs during pregnancy. The judge found that Stewart was charged under a statute that did not apply. (see "Fetal Abuse Isn't a Crime," April 1, 1988, *ABA Journal*, page 37.)

State Laws

Concern about pregnant women using drugs also has shifted to state legislatures. As of early June, about 20 different bills before the California legislature related in some way to pregnant women and drugs, according to Judith Rosen, a founder of California Advocates for Pregnant Women.

The bills' proposals ranged from establishing drug treatment programs for pregnant women to creating new criminal penalties, she said.

In Illinois, pending bills would establish drug treatment programs for pregnant women, and require hospitals to screen newborns of addicted mothers and report the results to the state child abuse agency.

An omnibus crime bill signed into law in Minnesota in June requires physicians to administer toxicology tests to pregnant women and newborns where there is evidence of illegal drug use. Positive results must be reported to local welfare agencies.

As many as 375,000 newborns a year may be affected by substance abuse in the United States, according to Dr. Ira Chasnoff, president of the National Association for Perinatal Addiction Research and Education (NAPARE).

Cocaine

One in 10 babies born in many urban areas has been exposed to cocaine in the womb.

Cocaine use puts the infant at least 10 times more at risk of crib death. It also can contribute to strokes while the fetus is in the womb or shortly after birth, and can cause other serious long-term health problems.

However, hospital- and community-based programs that offer treatment for drug addiction historically have excluded pregnant women.

Using existing criminal statutes to prosecute mothers for injuring their fetuses raises constitutional questions in view of the various abortion and privacy rulings by the Supreme Court.

Questions asked by the grand jury in the Green case suggested members were concerned about a woman's right to privacy and about criminalizing this type of behavior, said Paul Logli, the state's attorney who filed the charges.

Logli suggests that narrowly tailored laws be enacted. These laws should deal specifically with pregnant women using illegal drugs and should give some consideration to women who try to get drug treatment, he said.

Opponents of the new criminal prosecutions suggest that the

THREE WAYS TO DEAL WITH MATERNAL DRUG ABUSE

The **medical model** *starts with the premise of addiction being a disease but there is no consensus that totally supports this notion.*

The **social pathology/social deviance model** *attributes the addict's anti-social behaviors to environmental stresses and debilitating social forces—what one judge has called "rotten social background"—that is especially evident among minorities in the inner cities. The social pathology model recognizes the need for a wide-ranging attack on the problem which requires resources and compassion that are hard to come by. Faced with the enormity of the problem, criminalization of the behavior is seen by some as a "quick fix" solution.*

The **free will/personal choice model** *is based on the American majority opinion that people are free to choose to do right or wrong and are responsible for what they do.*

Sandra A. Garcia, Update, *November, 1989*

---

threat may drive pregnant women using illegal drugs away from health care facilities or may make them choose abortions.

Feminists say these types of prosecutions are unconstitutional and anti-women, and could lead down a slippery slope where pregnant women are prosecuted for consuming alcohol, smoking or failing to care properly for their fetuses.

"It's short-sighted and dangerous. . . and shows ignorance of addiction," said Lynn Paltrow of the ACLU's Reproductive Freedom Project. "These women don't hate their fetuses. They don't want to hurt their fetuses."

Every state has provisions requiring physicians and other health care workers to report child abuse and neglect, according to Walter Connolly Jr., a Detroit lawyer who represents hospitals. Two-thirds of the states impose both civil and criminal penalties on health care providers who fail to report child abuse.

Connolly suggests states should consider amending their statutes to include drug dependency at birth as a condition of abuse or neglect that must be reported.

But he worries about widespread felony prosecutions of pregnant women using illegal drugs.

"The role of the doctor would be as judge, jury and prosecutor. . . Every obstetrician and gynecologist will be in court testifying," he said.

On the civil side, there has been a growing recognition of

prenatal rights under tort law, according to Connolly. All 50 states recognize prenatal injury as a legitimate cause of action.

The question is whether liability for prenatal torts extends to pregnant women whose negligent actions caused injury to their subsequently born children.

In 1980, a Michigan appellate court allowed a son to sue his mother for negligently taking tetracycline while pregnant, causing his teeth to be brown.

Last November the Illinois Supreme Court denied a similar cause of action. The case involved a suit brought on behalf of a daughter against her mother for prenatal injuries that occurred during an automobile accident.

In reversing a lower court, the Illinois Supreme Court suggested such a cause of action would infringe upon a woman's right to privacy and bodily autonomy, pitting mother against fetus as legal adversaries from the moment of conception until birth.

The Illinois court said it would leave it up to the legislature to consider whether to recognize a legal duty of pregnant women to their developing fetuses.

Illinois State Sen. Richard Kelly said a child ought to have a right to take some kind of civil action against his or her mother for injuries due to illegal drug use while the woman was pregnant.

But Kelly, an abortion opponent, said he will not introduce a bill for fear such a law would lead to more abortions.

17   CRIME, PREGNANCY AND DRUGS

SOCIETY MUST CRIMINALIZE FETAL NEGLECT

Paul A. Logli

Paul A. Logli is the prosecuting attorney for Winnebago County, Rockford, Illinois. He believes that drug abusing pregnant mothers should be prosecuted.

Points to Consider:

1. Describe the substance of a "heartbreaking" letter the author received from a drug addicted mother.

2. What argument is made for criminal sanctions against drug addicted pregnant women?

3. How important are drug treatment and educational programs?

Paul A. Logli in a response to the editor's request for his position on the issue of criminal prosecution of substance abusing pregnant women, December, 1989.

The state must set out a definition of behavior which is so wanton in its disregard for human life and safety that persons engaging in it must be held responsible in the criminal courts.

Recently this office sought to bring charges against a 24-year-old mother as a result of the death of her two-day-old child. According to local medical authorities that death was directly related to the mother's use of cocaine during her pregnancy.

As events turned out, that prosecution was never advanced beyond the Winnebago County Grand Jury due to its decision not to indict the mother who had been previously charged on a police complaint. Thus this case was concluded without a chance to argue important issues before a judge or jury.

Social Controversy

In spite of this local setback, it is clear that the case has generated controversy and thought throughout the country. I have personally participated in discussions with numerous concerned individuals in New York, San Diego, Nashville, West Palm Beach, Chicago and Phoenix. It is apparent that the problem of children born either exposed or addicted to alcohol or drugs has become a difficult issue in practically every city and state. In most cases a child exposed or addicted will survive. That triumph, however, is tempered by continuing developmental problems, both physical and mental, that the child will face throughout his lifetime.

Adoptive Mother

I received a disturbing and heartbreaking letter from an adoptive mother in the Chicago suburbs. Her adopted child is now four years old and suffers from a multitude of physical problems ranging from cerebral palsy to bone deformities caused by the biological mother's alcohol and drug abuse during the pregnancy.

According to the letter writer, the biological mother was aware of the damage she was doing to her child while still in the womb and in spite of treatment at one of Chicago's prenatal centers for drug abusing pregnant women, the child was still damaged by the use of cocaine and other drugs throughout all stages of the pregnancy.

The letter writer states, "my heart breaks for my little girl, who though physically disabled, is intellectually intact as she watches her siblings run and play. She, even at this young age, wonders why she cannot! The truth is, she is a victim of a society that makes laws of convenience."

Unacceptable Behavior

Although it isn't convenient or simple, I have called upon the Legislature of the State of Illinois to set about the difficult task of first establishing that the protection of the health of our newborn has to be a priority in the medical, social and legal structures within our state. Secondly, having established this priority, they must work with experts in these areas to set out the boundaries of unacceptable behavior by pregnant women which may constitute a substantial threat to children who survive birth, but who are then captive to serious medical and educational disabilities.

Lastly, the state must set out a definition of behavior which is so wanton in its disregard for human life and safety that persons engaging in it must be held responsible in the criminal courts. I firmly believe criminalization of certain egregious behavior is an absolute requirement to go along with all of the social and medical planning which is also certainly needed.

We acknowledge that education, intervention, and the greater availability of drug treatment facilities for rich and poor alike is important in establishing a long-term solution to this problem. However, we know from our experience as prosecutors and in day-to-day life that people will not always do the right thing for the right reasons. Everyday we see persons who know the difference between right and wrong, but who are unwilling to conform their behavior to acceptable standards. Obviously there is no exception in the case of pregnant women.

Criminal Sanctions

Practically every high school in this nation has driver education courses, and there is no question that most drivers know the rules of the road. That, however, hasn't solved all of the highway safety problems that this society has encountered over the years. We are still required to conduct arrests of those people who, although knowing of the law, choose to disobey it. The analogy is no less accurate in regard to serious crime in our society, even when committed by drug addicts or pregnant

97

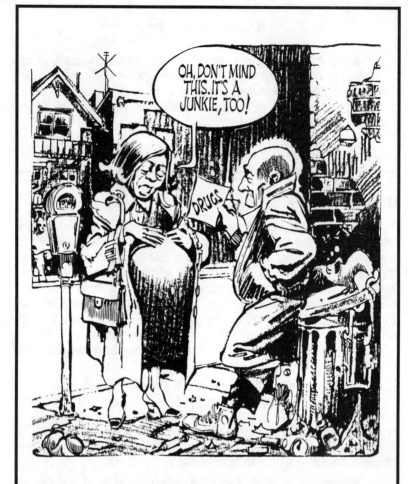

Illustration by David Seavey. Copyright 1990, *USA Today*. Reprinted with permission.

women.

We have decided to continue to play a key role in assisting our legislative leaders to draft appropriate legislation which, through criminal sanctions, discourages individuals from engaging in behavior harmful to the most innocent and defenseless members of our society, the newborn. We also encourage others, including the medical community, to assist the State in formulating and funding programs which will encourage and provide appropriate prenatal care and drug addiction treatment to anyone regardless of economic ability.

Only a comprehensive, well-funded effort which acknowledges the roles of intervention, prevention, education and deterrence can possibly accomplish the objective of guaranteeing the right of our children to a healthy birth.

18   CRIME, PREGNANCY AND DRUGS

USE TREATMENT, NOT PUNISHMENT

Ira J. Chasnoff

Ira J. Chasnoff, M.D. is President of the National Association for Perinatal Addiction, Research and Education, (NAPARE).

Points to Consider:

1. How has the medical community failed to deal with maternal drug abuse?

2. What is wrong with legal punishment of substance-abusing pregnant women?

3. Explain the role of the U.S. Congress on the issue of maternal drug abuse.

4. Why is access to health care vital in relation to the problem of substance abuse in pregnancy?

Ira J. Chasnoff, "President's Message", *Update,* November, 1989, page 2.

It is clear that the time and money spent on developing punitive intervention is time and money that could well be spent in developing treatment programs.

Treatment Programs, Not Punitive Interventions

It is clear that issues in substance abuse in pregnancy have entered the legal arena. Nowhere is this more evident than when we examine current newspapers and magazines reporting the trend in this country toward criminalization of substance abuse in pregnancy and punishment of substance-abusing pregnant women. This evolution into the current legal quagmire can trace its roots back to health care as it has been practiced in this country. As technology has invaded medical practice, physicians have become more distant from their patients relying on technology and pills to provide a cure.

Medical Failure

The art of history-taking has been lost in this evolution, so it is rare indeed that a physician will ask his patient about substance abuse or other lifestyle issues that can affect pregnancy outcome. The failure of the medical community to approach issues of substance abuse has resulted in misdiagnoses and emergency interventions required at a time of delivery. The cost in lives and dollars has been evident as this epidemic has spread and resulted in a growing level of frustration among both the medical and legal communities. This frustration has produced progressively more punitive measures aimed at substance-abusing pregnant women. It is clear, however, that as states become more punitive in their approach, the women that most need intervention are avoiding prenatal care.

Criminal Charges

This past summer, in Rockford, Illinois, a woman was charged with manslaughter and delivery of a controlled substance to a minor due to the death of her three-day-old infant following her cocaine use just prior to delivery. She came to the delivery room with premature labor. The infant died of anoxic brain damage, and an autopsy showed high levels of cocaine and cocaine metabolites in the body tissues. Following immediate coverage of this woman's arrest and incarceration, NAPARE's Cocaine Baby Helpline received record numbers of calls from women expressing fear if they should admit to their obstetricians their use of illicit drugs.

Reporting Laws

States with mandated reporting laws have overwhelmed their child protection and foster care systems with the large numbers of infants being reported. Minnesota recently enacted legislation that requires not only the reporting of a woman with a positive urine toxicology at delivery or a newborn infant with a positive urine toxicology at birth, but also the pregnant woman with a positive urine toxicology during the pregnancy. Accompanying this legislation is a realization that there are far too few treatment programs available to address the needs of the women reported through the system. Again, the pregnant, substance-abusing woman is being faced with the decision of risking incarceration by going for prenatal care. As laws are enacted in several states, it is clear that the time and money spent on developing punitive interventions is time and money that could well be spent in developing treatment programs.

Treatment

In a recent survey of 74 drug treatment programs in New York City, Dr. Wendy Chavkin from Columbia University, found that 54% of the treatment programs would not accept any pregnant women. 67% of the programs said they would not accept a pregnant woman on Medicaid, and 80% of the programs said they would not accept a pregnant woman on Medicaid who was using crack or cocaine. Thus, for all of New York City, less than 10 drug treatment programs are available for these pregnant women.

Congress has responded slowly to this crisis in treatment and appropriate intervention. In the Drug Omnibus Bill of 1988, funds were set aside for the development of demonstration programs for pregnant and postpartum women.

Grant procurement and awards were administered through the Federal Office for Substance Abuse Prevention (OSAP). Grant applications came from every part of the country. There were $137 million of grant applications; however, only 4.5 million dollars were available to be awarded, far short of the needed amount. Congress is currently looking at new legislation which would expand these treatment programs and would provide

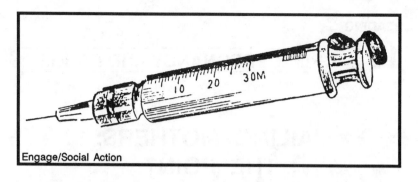
Engage/Social Action

resources for referral and consultation for both the public and the professional communities. State-blocked grants will continue to focus on needs of the pregnant, substance-abusing woman and her child. However, the real success of any program will rely on community organizations. It is becoming increasingly evident that physicians, nurses, social workers, and other health care professionals must take the leadership in providing interventions and treatment for pregnant women, as well as developing coordinated multidisciplinary models for prenatal and postpartum care.

Health Care Access

The issues involved in substance abuse in pregnancy are not isolated issues of substance abuse per se, but rather issues of access to health care. Non-punitive supportive programs must be put in place to provide the necessary treatment structure within the community. It is hoped that members of NAPARE in communities throughout the country can provide the leadership for the development of these programs.

The current situation reminds me of the story of the three fishermen. It was a sunny, spring day and three long-time friends were fishing along a swiftly moving river. Suddenly, they saw a baby floating down the river. The first fisherman ran into the river and pulled the baby out. They looked at each other quizzically, wondering where this baby had come from. They turned back and looked up stream and saw another baby, and then another. And soon hundreds of babies were floating by caught in the rapid movement of the stream. The three fisherman waded out to the middle of the river and pulled baby after baby out of the water. One of the fishermen suddenly ran out of the river and began running upstream. His two friends yelled at him to come back and help; "Where are you going? We're pulling babies out of the water." He looked back quickly and continued upstream. "You two can stay here and pull babies out of the river," he said, "I'm going upstream to find out who is throwing the babies in."

19 CRIME, PREGNANCY AND DRUGS

JAILING MOTHERS: THE POINT

Charles Krauthammer

Charles Krauthammer is a nationally syndicated political columnist and writes weekly for The New Republic *magazine.*

Points to Consider:

1. Describe the meaning of the "bio-underclass".

2. How well might punishment of mothers work to solve the problem of cocaine babies?

3. What role should treatment programs play?

4. Why is "locking up" mothers described as a workable option?

Taking custody of the child unfortunately but necessarily means taking custody of the mother.

Crack Cocaine

The newest horror produced by the crack epidemic, particularly in the inner city, is a bio-underclass, a generation of cocaine babies, physically damaged and mentally retarded, whose future prospects are, effectively, biologically destroyed at birth.

Government

Can government really do anything about women so controlled by cocaine that they risk horrible damage to their babies by doing crack during pregnancy? A new burden for inner-city hospitals is cocaine babies abandoned by mothers who simply leave the hospital after delivery and never come back. Cocaine may be the most effective destroyer of the maternal instinct ever found.

The other voice of despair says that until the government solves the drug problem as a whole, it cannot hope to solve the problem of cocaine babies. This, too, may be true, but it is irresponsible as well as cruel not to try to save some babies pending solution of the larger drug problem. But how?

Punishment

Several jurisdictions have tried criminal prosecution. Three weeks ago a judge in Florida found a 23-year-old mother guilty of criminally conveying cocaine to her (unborn) child. This case followed a string of legal failures, the most prominent of which occurred in Winnebago County, Ill., where a grand jury refused to indict Melanie Green of involuntary manslaughter for killing her fetus with cocaine.

The jury was probably right. Current legislation, never intended for the contingency of cocaine babies, is too vague to sustain such a conviction. Moreover, criminal sanctions probably won't work. If concern for the child is no deterrent to a pregnant crack addict, concern for the justice system is hardly a better one.

One rationale for not prosecuting cocaine mothers is entirely fatuous, however. Leave it to the local American Civil Liberties Union to offer it. It praised the Green jury for refusing "to criminalize and punish a pregnant woman who was herself a victim and who had already lost her child."

The number of middle-class whites so addicted to rights and so enamored of victimhood is shocking. It is one thing to let the homeless mentally ill die with their rights in the streets of America. You might, if you stretch it, say that these adults are destroying themselves; the state has no business interfering in people's privacy.

But how can you maintain the fiction that a woman who does crack during pregnancy is protected from state intrusion because she too is engaged in a self-regarding act? The hospital wards filled with these tormented infants refute the proposition.

Treatment

The liberal answer, of course, is not to punish these women but to treat them. But that assumes that they will accept treatment. In the District of Columbia, prenatal care is free and the city has made an effort to bring pregnant woman in for help. Yet, at Greater Southeast Community Hospital, 25 to 30 drug-abusing women show up every month for delivery.

"A person who is addicted to drugs has another priority," explains Pamela Robinson, a social worker at the hospital. "The unborn child is not a priority." Care for these mothers, says Robinson, "is available, and they are aware of it, but they are not seeking care."

The other problem with treatment for crack addiction is that we do not have the slightest idea how to go about it. Douglas Besharov, a scholar at the American Enterprise Institute who has studied the drug problem for 20 years, concludes that, "there is almost no evidence of our ability to deliver a successful drug treatment program to people."

Heroin successes are due either to the development of blocking drugs (like methadone) or to programs with a charismatic leader who uniquely engages the participants. Otherwise? "There's no proof that this stuff makes a difference," concludes Besharov.

Custody

Jeaneen Grey Eagle, who runs an alcohol treatment program at the Pine Ridge Reservation in South Dakota, tells the *New York Times* that her tribe once locked up a pregnant woman

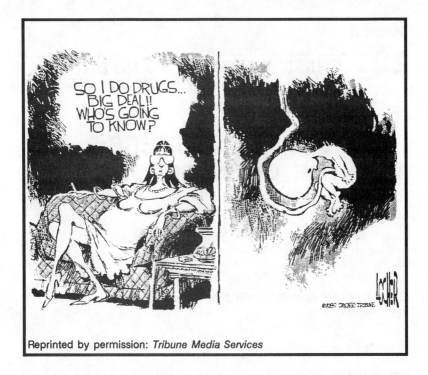

who could not stop drinking. She supports such action.

So do I. The choice is simple. We can either do nothing, or we can pass laws saying that any pregnant woman who takes cocaine during pregnancy will be sent until delivery to some not uncomfortable, secure location where she will be allowed everything except the liberty to leave, or to take drugs.

Protection

We should do this not as punishment, nor as vengeance, nor even for deterrence, but purely for the protection of the soon-to-be-born child. Taking custody of the child unfortunately but necessarily means taking custody of the mother.

This is no solution to the mother's drug problem. But it is a solution to the baby's. There might be a better solution fairer to both, but no one can find it. And until we do, the bio-underclass grows.

JAILING MOTHERS:
THE COUNTERPOINT

Ellen Goodman

Ellen Goodman is a nationally syndicated columnist and writes for the Boston Globe.

Points to Consider:

1. Why do most "cocaine babies" never get over their problems?

2. Describe the syndrome of those who are born addicted.

3. What is the relation between anger and punishment?

4. Describe the public debate that is taking place.

5. Why is jailing pregnant women a bad policy?

How ironic to spend money jailing mothers while others who seek help are being turned away, because there is no room at the treatment center.

Cocaine Babies

The poster on the hospital wall doesn't waste any words. Over the picture of a baby it says: "Some of the people who take cocaine during pregnancy never get over it."

This is more than a public service warning to pregnant women. It's also the bottom line from the research done on the cocaine babies. Most never get over it.

Treatment Program

On this summer morning in the clinic at Northwestern University's medical school hospital, Dan Griffith is seeing some children brought in for long-term follow-up as part of a project on pregnant substance abusers and their babies under the umbrella of the National Association for Perinatal Research and Education. Carefully, the burly and gentle psychologist watches two-year-old Stacy as she uses blocks and crayons and walks along the string on the floor.

It takes a trained eye to identify the symptoms in Stacy. She is among what Griffith calls "the best of the worst". In this treatment program, they see the mothers who came for treatment, the babies who survived, the toddlers who have had attention.

Born Addicted

But he knows well the syndrome of those born addicted. Newborns who go from sleeping to screaming, and cannot maintain the state of quiet alertness during which bonding and learning take place. Toddlers who can't tolerate stimulation. School children who are easily distracted and more easily frustrated.

These would not be easy children for the strongest families. Even the "best of the worst" have started a life permanently imprinted, scarred, with neurological damage.

How many such kids are there? Last year, the association found that a staggering 11 percent of babies born in 36 hospitals in 1988 had mothers who used illegal drugs while they were pregnant. That's some 375,000 mothers.

Anger and Frustration

"The question I am asked most often," said Griffith, "is how do you work with mothers who have done that to their kids?" It's less a question than a judgment that springs up easily in an

109

atmosphere of public frustration at drugs and anger at the irresponsibility of a pregnant woman.

Lately, that anger has turned to a passion for punishment. Not far from here, a Rockford woman named Melanie Green was put on trial last May before a grand jury for manslaughter in the death of her addicted newborn. This summer in Florida, Jennifer Johnson was convicted of delivering drugs to the recipient in her womb. Other courts, seeking to protect the fetus before birth, have moved pregnant women to jail until delivery.

Public Debate

The public debate over pregnant drug abusers has turned frequently into an argument over the rights of the fetus versus the rights of the pregnant woman. Those who hold a front-row seat at the devastation of these cocaine babies, who know that drug abuse is the primary cause of infant mortality, have the greatest right to judge these pregnant women. Yet they are more likely to view the argument over rights and the passion to lock-'em-up as a great diversion.

"If you jail one woman, the only lesson you teach women is to stay out of the prenatal health care system," says Dr. Ira Chasnoff, head of the perinatal association. The lesson he wants to deliver to these mothers is quite the opposite: Come in for health care. Now.

Chasnoff believes there is no shortcut for the kinds of prenatal identification and treatment that his group has been developing.

Jailing Women

As for jailing pregnant women, he runs through the real life scenario. If we jail women until delivery in a mythical drug-free prison, do we then send them and their babies back to the same streets? Do we, on the other hand, take the children away from their mothers and put them into the beleaguered foster care system? And will we jail those children again when they are 16, pregnant and strung-out?

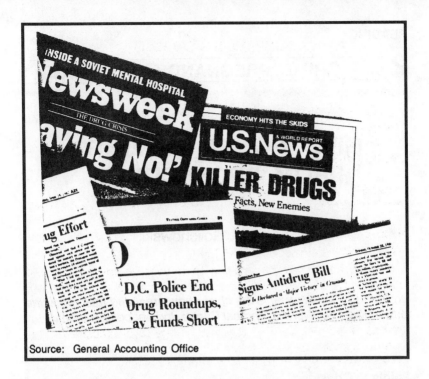

INSIDE A SOVIET MENTAL HOSPITAL

Newsweek

THE DRUG CRISIS

aying No!'

ECONOMY HITS THE SKIDS

U.S.News
& WORLD REPORT

KILLER DRUGS
Facts, New Enemies

ug Effort

D.C. Police End
Drug Roundups,
'ay Funds Short

Signs Antidrug Bill
ture Is Declared a 'Major Victory' in Crusade

Source: General Accounting Office

The most popular proposal that drug czar William Bennett has made is for more jail space, but those who work in the fallout of the drug world shake their heads at this. Their impulse is not to lock-'em-up. When they talk about mothers and babies, the issue is not whose rights are violated but what works.

And the irony doesn't escape their notice. How ironic to spend money jailing mothers while others who seek help are being turned away, because there is no room at the treatment center.

GIVE WOMEN IMMUNITY FROM PROSECUTION

Alan M. Golichowski

Dr. Alan M. Golichowski is the chief of maternal and fetal medicine at the Indiana University Medical Center, Indianapolis, Indiana.

Points to Consider:

1. Explain the relationship between drugs and children.

2. How prevalent is cocaine use by pregnant mothers?

3. What steps should be taken to solve this problem?

4. Why are no further studies needed on the effect of drug use during pregnancy?

5. When should addicted pregnant women be given immunity from prosecution?

Alan M. Golichowski in testimony before the Senate Committee on Labor and Human Resources, October 9, 1989.

The long-term outcome will be better for their infants if addicted pregnant women are given immunity from criminal prosecution if they seek treatment.

This time is exceedingly important because of two great forces threatening the well-being of pregnant women and children. The first of these forces is the great tragedy of infant mortality. The second is the overwhelming problem of drugs in the United States in general and the specific devastating impact that drugs are having on future generations of Americans. The use of cocaine, crack, heroin, alcohol, speed, and a multitude of street drugs that are taken during pregnancy cause a lifetime of devastating effects for children born under these circumstances.

Drugs and Children

There are several hundred drugs, that if taken during pregnancy, can have devastating effects on the child for many years to come after their birth. Think of diethylstilbestrol. When a small amount of this drug is taken during pregnancy, it causes a lifetime of mental retardation for a child. We are now confronted with a drug which when taken in pregnancy has even more disastrous effects on the child.

Cocaine is now used by literally thousands of pregnant women. This highly addictive drug now further destroys future generations of Americans. In my opinion what we need are comprehensive programs of education, detection, and early treatment of mothers-to-be who are affected by this drug.

In the past six months my colleagues and I have had to deal with pregnancies in which the brain of the fetus has been destroyed and turned to liquid by strokes caused by the use of cocaine. We have cared for women whose children will have limited use of their arms and legs because of prenatal damage to their nervous systems by cocaine. And we have cared for women whose children are spared these problems only to have lives plagued by learning disabilities. We are having to deal with problems such as these with ever increasing frequency.

National Effort Needed

It is my hope that people hear the plea from obstetricians and maternal fetal specialists throughout the entire United States that we must attack and bring into submission, the problem of crack in pregnancy with every possible approach. We desperately need the efforts of national leaders along with the efforts of health professionals, to deal with this problem in a humane and comprehensive way.

We do not need any further studies on the effect of alcohol and cocaine use during pregnancy. Every study concludes that the effects are disastrous for the fetus. What we need are programs to prevent the use of these drugs in pregnancies. It is my sincere hope and plea that a major national effort can come forth that will attack the problem of preventing cocaine use in pregnancy. The problem can be stated most clearly. If a woman does not drink nor take drugs during pregnancy she does not have a crack baby or a child with fetal alcohol syndrome. It is a tragedy for any woman to become an addict of either alcohol or cocaine. It is an extreme tragedy when the child that she is carrying will have the lifetime consequences of her addiction. We simply must protect unborn children.

Indiana

We have the statistics to clearly delineate the problem of crack use in pregnancy in the State of Indiana and the City of Indianapolis. We do not have the whole story. We do know that the problem here is similar to that reported in other parts of the United States. Some evidence of the magnitude of the problem in our community of Indianapolis is revealed in a study that was conducted a year ago by Dr. Beth Norman, Dr. Richard Hansell, and Dr. Michael Evans of the Indiana University School of Medicine. These investigators found that three percent of women in labor had traces of cocaine in their urine. Seven percent of women who were seen for placental abruption, or separation of the placenta from the uterus before delivery, which is known to be related to the use of cocaine, had positive urine tests for cocaine; 25% of these women gave a history of cocaine use. I wish to emphasize that this study was completed a year ago and that I personally believe the problem is much more pronounced at present. If our community is similar to those whose experience has been reported, the current prevalence should be twice as high.

Prosecution and Prenatal Care

One of my personal concerns is that in this war on drugs you

114

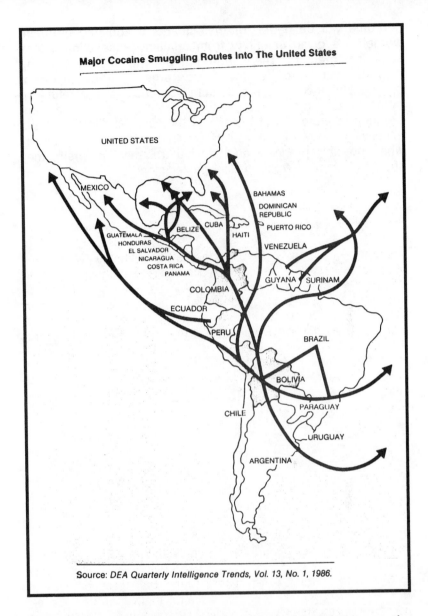

Major Cocaine Smuggling Routes Into The United States

UNITED STATES

MEXICO

BAHAMAS

DOMINICAN REPUBLIC

PUERTO RICO

BELIZE

CUBA

HAITI

GUATEMALA
HONDURAS
EL SALVADOR
NICARAGUA
COSTA RICA
PANAMA

VENEZUELA

COLOMBIA

GUYANA SURINAM

ECUADOR

PERU

BRAZIL

BOLIVIA

PARAGUAY

CHILE

URUGUAY

ARGENTINA

Source: *DEA Quarterly Intelligence Trends, Vol. 13, No. 1, 1986.*

consider very carefully the legal effects of legislation on the practice of medicine and on preventive health care. I am deeply concerned that if physicians are required to report cocaine use during pregnancy to legal authorities and this results in criminal prosecution of the pregnant woman, that many pregnant women will no longer seek prenatal care. If a pregnant woman is threatened by criminal prosecution when she seeks prenatal care, then the effect will be to drive women who are addicted to drugs away from the health care system, and the long-term effect will result in more crack babies, more fetal alcohol babies, and increased infant mortality. I believe that the long-term outcome will be better for their infants if addicted pregnant women are given immunity from criminal prosecution if they seek treatment for their addiction by immediately entering prenatal care and treatment programs. Without a doubt pregnant women who are addicted to cocaine and refuse to come in for prenatal care and refuse to enter a treatment program to protect the fetus should be dealt with vigorously and effectively. However, if addicts would come forth immediately when possibly pregnant and enter a treatment program, they should be immune from criminal prosecution.

22   CRIME, PREGNANCY AND DRUGS

DON'T DECRIMINALIZE DRUG DEALING TO INFANTS

Stephen Goldsmith

Stephen Goldsmith is the prosecutor for Marion County, Indiana. He previously served on the Indiana Attorney General's Advisory Board on Missing and Exploited Children.

Points to Consider:

1. In order to prosecute a drug-using pregnant mother for child abuse, what kind of evidence is needed?

2. What people are in favor of decriminalizing drug dealing to infants?

3. How is the "prosecution medical model" defined?

4. What role should prosecutors and medical professionals play in solving the problem of maternal drug abuse?

5. Why is there nothing inconsistent with the concepts of punishment and treatment?

Stephen Goldsmith in testimony before the Senate Committee on Labor and Human Resources, October 9, 1989.

Those who argue against prosecution essentially argue for decriminalizing drug dealing to infants, which obviously sends the wrong message.

I have previously served as the only District Attorney appointed to the Attorney General's Advisory Board on Missing and Exploited Children and currently am chairman of a joint task force of drug-affected babies set up by the National Center for the Prosecution of Child Abuse and the Center for Local Prosecution of Drug Offenses. . .

Range of Prosecutorial Choices

An Indiana prosecutor has several choices. Evidence of a controlled substance in the child's or mother's blood system might be adequate proof of possession by the mother, allowing for prosecution.

A positive test on the baby could lead to a charge of delivering a controlled substance because it is inevitable that the drugs were delivered through the umbilical cord momentarily after birth. A mother who is nursing and on cocaine will also be delivering the substance to the baby. A charge of Neglect of a Dependent might also be possible.

Additionally, the prosecutor or the welfare department could bring a Child in Need of Services (CHINS) petition based on the addiction of the child.

Finally Indiana might consider passing laws making the use of drugs illegal or extending more protection to the fetus. In Indiana today the only law that would clearly protect the fetus makes it a crime to kill a fetus. Indiana, of course, could add other crimes. This state was one of the first to pass a law making it illegal to drive with a controlled substance in the blood stream. We did this while I was Chairman of the Governor's Task Force Against Drunk Driving. This per se law (it is illegal per se; the amount is irrelevant as is the impairment) would serve as a model for possible legislation concerning drug use during pregnancy.

A Proposal for a Comprehensive Response

The purpose of a legislative and programmatic response should be to increase the chances that the mother will reduce or eliminate her drug use as early as possible. The question then becomes whether prosecutor involvement is constructive. With the enormous number of drug babies existing now nationally, one could easily claim that it is difficult to see how our involvement could make the situation worse.

However, a more thorough response indicates a possible middle ground. A joint medical/legal task force in Indianapolis is investigating a wide range of responses. Isolated prosecutions of mothers whose children are addicted might be appropriate, but so long as they are relatively limited in number, they will have little effect. Undervalued in the national dialogue is the effect of a well-publicized prosecution in emphasizing to the public generally (the casual user) the wrongfulness of the conduct. Those who argue against prosecution essentially argue for decriminalizing drug dealing to infants, which obviously sends the wrong message.

Hospital and Medical Response

Prenatal and pre-delivery urine tests must include, for medical purposes, a test for cocaine. A high-level medical advisory group should accumulate information and publish findings. . .

If the medical community is unwilling to approach the solution in this manner, then cities, states, or the federal government should consider mandated testing of newborns.

Similarly, the postnatal effects of cocaine may be less clear, but research reflects problems with infant motor skills and spatial orientation, and other difficulties. Testing of the baby and the mother at birth should occur for purposes of pediatric involvement. Mothers who breastfeed should be dissuaded from using cocaine and should be tested on a regular basis.

In Indiana, the positive test at delivery of the child and perhaps the mother require notification to the Department of Public Welfare under mandatory child abuse reporting laws. Such a report would not be different in type than other abuse reports now made by hospitals based on lesser levels of evidence.

The Child Protective Service or Prosecutor Response

I recommend a combined approach with the hospital pediatrician and the prosecutor. Under this approach, a positive maternal cocaine test would lead to an agreement between the state, the mother, and the medical provider. It would provide for a medical regimen (i.e., a discharge agreement which would require treatment and urine tests over a period of time plus increased pediatric involvement. The prosecutor would agree to withhold charges if the mother successfully completes terms of the agreement.

A model for this approach exists in this city in the area of educational neglect and truancy. At the request of the schools we send letters to parents of grade school children who are regularly absent telling the parents to reach an accord with the school counselors, or we will prosecute for educational neglect. This procedure has been effective.

Necessary Responses and the Problems

Prenatal Care

a. Testing

A critical goal is to pursue a prosecution/medical model that encourages and not discourages treatment. Such a result is more probably accomplished postnatally. Prenatal care should require cocaine testing for purposes of medical attention. The positive results would not necessarily need to be reported (at least during a research and evaluation period).

If a mother tested positive early in her pregnancy, then treatment and intensive counselling could occur. Indeed, a district attorney could establish a policy for post-delivery prosecutions that provides a benefit to those who have sought prenatal care. Prosecutions or agreements with mothers concerning medical neglect or delivery of cocaine to the infant could lead to reduced charges or sentences for the mother who obtained prenatal care. Thus the prosecutor in a refined policy could encourage prenatal testing through subsequent lesser prosecution.

b. AFDC

Similarly, we need to address the larger question of access to and availability of prenatal care. The Senate should evaluate the possibility of moving mandated AFDC eligibility back to the time when a doctor determines that a pregnancy exists. Such a decision would encourage mothers to receive medical attention and would allow for a range of services and interventions that do not now occur. . .

Additionally, I spend considerable time involved in the national effort to collect child support. Fathers should be responsible from the point of conception for the care of the children. Some of the costs would be offset by child support collection, and the early intervention with the father would not only yield short-term collections, but would improve long-term collections through increased paternity establishments and knowledge of the location of the father. Also an earlier enforcement strategy would force the father to pay attention to the consequences of his actions and the possible consequences of the mother's cocaine use.

Finally, the fetus deserves at least that much protection from our society from this early intervention.

Treatment

The most significant problem that exists is the absence of adequate treatment and the pronounced absence of evaluations of successful treatment strategy. Treatment, which would be a condition of an enforced agreement by a prosecutor, must be available. In this community where the state invests little in drug treatment, assistance for poorer families is barely available, and then only after long waits.

Medical benefits should be expanded to include post-delivery substance abuse treatment when the mother tests positive for drugs. There is considerable confusion in Indiana whether such coverage is available under current law, with the general opinion that it is not. To turn the cocaine-using mother and child back out into their community with no treatment resources not only harms the child but inevitably increases the costs to society.

Conclusion

There is nothing inconsistent with punishment and treatment. The research that our Task Force Against Drunk Driving heard presented in testimony clearly reflected that successful alcohol intervention was as likely to succeed if the person were forced to counselling by the justice system as if he entered on his own. Therefore the club of prosecution should be used to force treatment.

ASSAULTING THE POOR

Katha Pollitt

Katha Pollit wrote the following comments in The Nation *magazine. She is currently working on a collection of essays on women's issues.*

Points to Consider:

1. How is punishing pregnant drug abusers described as a "contradiction"?

2. Why is the concern over pregnant drug abusers called an "assault on the poor"?

3. Why is concern for the fetus not helping children?

4. How is the book, *The Broken Cord* by Michael Dorris, described?

All over the country, pregnant women who use illegal drugs and/or alcohol are targeted by the criminal justice system. They are "preventively detained" by judges who give out jail sentences for minor crimes that would ordinarily result in probation or a fine; charged with child abuse or neglect (although by law the fetus is not a child) and threatened with manslaughter charges should they miscarry; and placed under court orders not to drink, although drinking is not a crime and does not invariably (or even usually) result in birth defects. . .

What's going on here? Right now the hot area in the developing issue of "fetal rights" is the use of drugs and alcohol during pregnancy. We've all seen the nightly news reports of inner-city intensive care units overflowing with crack babies, of Indian reservations where one in four children is said to be born physically and mentally stunted by fetal alcohol syndrome (FAS) or the milder, but still serious, fetal alcohol effect. We've read the front page stories reporting studies that suggest staggering rates of drug use during pregnancy (11 percent, according to *The New York Times,* or 370,000 women per year) and the dangers of even moderate drinking during pregnancy. . .

Punitive Approach

Critics of the punitive approach to pregnant drug and alcohol users point out the ironies inherent in treating a public health concern as a matter for the criminal justice system: the contradiction, for instance, of punishing addicted women when most drug treatment programs refuse to accept pregnant women. Indeed, Jennifer Johnson, a Florida woman who was the first person convicted after giving birth to a baby who tested positive for cocaine, had sought treatment and been turned away. (In her case the charge was delivering drugs to a minor.) The critics point out that threats of jail or the loss of their kids may drive women away from prenatal care and hospital deliveries, and that almost all the women affected so far have been poor and black or latino, without private doctors to protect them (in Florida, nonwhite women are ten times as likely to be reported for substance abuse as white women, although rates of drug use are actually higher for whites).

These are all important points. But they leave unchallenged the notion of fetal rights themselves. What we really ought to be asking is, how have we come to see women as the major threat to the health of their newborns, and the womb as the most dangerous place a child will ever inhabit? The list of dangers to the fetus is, after all, very long; the list of dangers to children even longer. Why does maternal behavior, a relatively small piece of the total picture, seem such an urgent matter, while much more important factors—that one in five pregnant women receive no prenatal care at all, for instance—attract so little attention? Here are some of the strands that make up the current tangle of fetal rights.

The Assault on the Poor

It would be pleasant to report that the aura of crisis surrounding crack and FAS babies—the urge to do something, however unconstitutional or cruel, that suddenly pervades society, from judge's bench to chic dinner party to 7 o'clock news—was part of a massive national campaign to help women have healthy, wanted pregnancies and healthy babies. But significantly, the current wave of concern is not occurring in that context. Judges order pregnant addicts to jail, but they don't order drug treatment programs to accept them, or Medicaid, which pays for heroin treatment, to cover crack addiction—let alone order landlords not to evict them, or obstetricians to take uninsured women as patients, or the federal government to fund fully the Women, Infants, and Children supplemental feeding program, which reaches only two-thirds of those who are eligible. The policies that have underwritten maternal and infant health in most of the industrialized West since World War II—a national health service, paid maternity leave, direct payments to mothers, government-funded day care, home health visitors for new mothers, welfare payments that reflect the cost of living—are still regarded in the United States by even the most liberal as hopeless causes, and by everyone else as budget-breaking giveaways to the undeserving-pie-in-the-sky items from a mad socialist's wish list.

The focus on maternal behavior allows the government to appear to be concerned about babies without having to spend any money, change any priorities or challenge any vested interests. As with crime, as with poverty, a complicated, multifaceted problem is construed as a matter of freely chosen individual behavior. We have crime because we have lots of bad people, poverty because we have lots of lazy people (Republican version) or lots of pathological people (Democratic version), and tiny, sickly, impaired babies because we have lots of women who just don't give a damn.

Once the problem has been defined as original sin, coercion and punishment start to look like hardheaded and common-sensical answers. Thus, syndicated columnist and *New Republic* intellectual Charles Krauthammer proposes locking up pregnant drug users en masse. Never mind the impracticality of the notion — suddenly the same Administration that refuses to pay for drug treatment and prenatal care is supposed to finance all that plus nine months of detention for hundreds of thousands of women a year. . .

The Privileged Status of the Fetus

Pro-choice activists rightly argue that anti-abortion and fetal-rights advocates grant fetuses more rights than women. A point less often made is that they grant fetuses more rights than two-year-olds — the right, for example, to a safe, healthy place to live. . .

Although concern for the fetus may look like a way of helping children, it is actually, in a funny way, a substitute for it. It is an illusion to think that by "protecting" the fetus from its mother's behavior we have insured a healthy birth, a healthy infancy or a healthy childhood, and that the only insurmountable obstacle for crack babies is prenatal exposure to crack.

It is no coincidence that we are obsessed with pregnant women's behavior at the same time that children's health is declining, by virtually any yardstick one chooses. Take general well-being: in constant dollars, welfare payments are now about two-thirds the 1965 level. Take housing: thousands of children are now growing up in homeless shelters and welfare hotels. Even desperately alcoholic women bear healthy babies two-thirds of the time. Will two-thirds of today's homeless kids emerge unscathed from their dangerous and lead-permeated environments? Take access to medical care: inner-city hospitals are closing all over the country, millions of kids have no health insurance and most doctors refuse uninsured or Medicaid patients. Even immunization rates are down: whooping cough and measles are on the rise. . .

Women's Duties

The *Broken Cord*, Michael Dorris's much-praised memoir of his adopted FAS child, Adam, is a textbook example of the way in which all these social trends come together — and the largely uncritical attention the book has received shows how seductive a pattern they make. Dorris has nothing but contempt for Adam's birth mother. Perhaps it is asking too much of human nature to expect him to feel much sympathy for her. He has witnessed, in the most intimate and heartbreaking way, the damage her alcoholism did, and seen the ruin of his every hope for Adam, who is deeply retarded. But why is his anger directed only at her? Here was a seriously alcoholic woman, living on an Indian reservation where heavy drinking is a way of life, along with poverty, squalor, violence, despair and powerlessness, where, one might even say, a kind of racial suicide is taking place, with liquor as the weapon of choice. Adam's mother, in fact, died two years after his birth from drinking antifreeze. . .

"People are always talking about women's duties to others," said Lyn Paltrow, the A.C.L.U. lawyer who successfully led the Pamela Rae Stewart defense, "as though women were not the chief caregivers in this society." But no one talks about women's duty of care to themselves. A pregnant addict or alcoholic needs to get help for herself. She's not just potentially ruining someone else's life. She's ruining her own life.

"Why isn't her own life important? Why don't we care about her?"

Examining Counterpoints

This activity may be used as an individual study guide for students in libraries and resource centers or as a discussion catalyst in small group classroom discussions.

Criminal Sanctions: The Point

Society is not responsible for maternal drug abuse. People are responsible for their own decisions. Drug-abusing pregnant women should be locked up and only permitted to ingest things that will not damage their babies. After birth, babies should be placed in foster care or placed for adoption, if the mother cannot prove she is free from drug habits. Any mothers who damage their babies by abusing drugs during pregnancy should be prosecuted and face prison if the harm inflicted is serious. Pregnant women who abuse their babies with drugs of any kind are criminals. Only tough criminal sanctions will deter pregnant mothers from their destructive drug habits.

Criminal Sanctions: The Counterpoint

Criminal sanctions will not stop the problems of maternal drug abuse. This will create fear among pregnant substance-abusing mothers. They will then not tell their doctors and medical authorities that they desperately need help and treatment. Society must provide treatment, not punishment, for drug-abusing pregnant mothers. There are very few treatment centers and programs for maternal drug abuse. Society must provide these important educational and treatment facilities to effectively deal with the issue of maternal drug abuse.

Guidelines

1. Social issues are usually complex, but often problems become oversimplified in political debates and discussion. Usually a polarized version of social conflict does not adequately represent the diversity of views that surround social conflicts.

2. Examine the counterpoints above. Then write down other possible interpretations of this issue than the two arguments stated in the counterpoints above.

BIBLIOGRAPHY

DRUG ADDICTED BABIES

Aase, Jon M. "The Fetal Alcohol Syndrome in American Indians": A High Risk Group. *Neurobehavioral Toxicology and Teratology* 3: 153-156, 1981.

American Medical Association, Council on Scientific Affairs. "Fetal Effects of Maternal Alcohol Use," *Journal of the American Medical Association* 249 (18): 2517-2521, 1983.

Anonymous. "Mother's Experience with Fetal Alcohol Effects," *Lakota Times*, 3/12/86.

Brody, Jane E. "An Estimated 50,000 Babies Born Last Year Suffered from Prenatal Alcohol Exposure," *New York Times*, 1/15/86.

_____. "Any Drink During Pregnancy May Be One Too Many, Latest Research into Fetal Alcohol Syndrome shows," *Minneapolis Star Tribune*, 2/23/86.

_____. "Widespread Abuse of Drugs by Pregnant Women," *New York Times*, 8/30/88.

Center for Science in the Public Interest. "S. 2047, H.R. 4441. A Bill to Require Health Warning Labels on All Alcoholic Beverage Containers" [leaflet]. 1501 Sixteenth Street, NW, Washington, DC 20036.

Chambers, Marcia. "Are Fetal Rights Equal to Infants'?" *New York Times*, 11/16/86.

Chasnoff, I. J. Perinatal Effects of Cocaine. *Contemporary Obstetrics and Gynecology* 1987: 29: 163-170.

Chasnoff I. J. Drugs and Women: Establishing a Standard of Care. *Annals Of The New York Academy of Medicine*, to be published.

Chavez, Gilberto, Jose Cordero and Jose Becerra. "Leading Major Congenital Malformations Among Minority Groups in the United States, 1981-1986," Centers for Disease Control: Morbidity and Morality Weekly Special Edition 37 (SS-3): 17-24, 1988.

Davis, Janet Haggerty, and W. A. Frost. "Fetal Alcohol Syndrome: A Challenge for the Community Health Nurse," *Journal of Community Health Nursing* 1 (2): 99-110, 1984.

Department of the Interior. Alcohol and Drug Abuse in BIA Schools [unpublished] (Washington, DC: Bureau of Indian Affairs, June 1982).

Enloe, Cortez F. "How Alcohol Affects the Developing Fetus," *Nutrition Today* 15 (5): 12-15, 1980.

Eyler, F. "The Cocaine Connection". Presented at 6th Annual Parent Care Conference. September 21-24, 1989, Chicago.

Forbes, Ronald. "Alcohol-related Birth Defects," *Public Health, London* 98: 231-241, 1984.

Fox, S. H., C. Brown, A. M. Koontz, and S. S. Kessel. "Perceptions of Risks of Smoking and Heavy Drinking During Pregnancy: 1985 NHIS Findings," *Public Health Reports* 102 (1): 73-79, 1987.

Goleman, Daniel. "Lasting Costs for Child Are Found from a Few Early Drinks," *New York Times*, 2/16/89.

_____. "Major Personality Study Finds That Traits Are Mostly Inherited," *New York Times*, 12/2/86.

Graham, J. M. "Alcohol Consumption and Pregnancy." In Marios, M., ed., *Prevention of Congenital Malformations* (New York: A. R. Liss, 1983).

_____, and A. M. Cooper. Alcohol Use and World Cultures: *A Comprehensive Bibliography of Anthropological Sources* (Toronto: Addiction Research Foundation, 1981).

Iber, Frank L. "Fetal Alcohol Syndrome," *Nutrition Today* 15 (5): 3-11, 1980.

Issues and Answers in Perinatal and Neonatal Care. First Annual Symposium of the Perinatal Improvement Network, held at Davis, Ca., May 1988. Davis, University of California.

Jessup, M., and J. R. Green. "Treatment of the Pregnant Alcohol-Dependent Woman," *Journal of Psychoactive Drugs* 19 (2): 193-203, 1987.

Lamanna, Michael. "Alcohol Related Birth Defects: Implications for Education," *Journal of Drug Education* 12 (2): 113-123, 1982.

Landers, A. "Disposition Largely a Matter of Genes?" syndicated column, May 1988.

Landry, M. Smith D.: Crack, Smoking Cocaine. *San Francisco Medicine* 1987. Jan. 30, 31 and 42.

Larson, C. P., Pless I. B.: Risk Factors for Injury in a 3-Year-Old Birth Cohort. *American Journal of Disabled Children* 1988. 142:1052-1057.

Lele, Amol S. "Fetal Alcohol Syndrome: Other Effects of Alcohol on Pregnancy," *New York State Journal of Medicine,* pp. 1225-1227, July 1982.

Lewin, Tamar. "When Courts Take Charge of the Unborn," *New York Times,* 1/19/89.

Madden, J. S., Payne I. F., Miller S: Maternal Cocaine Abuse and Effect on The Newborn. *Pediatrics* 1986: 77:209-211.

Marbury, Marian D., S. Linn, R. Monson et al. "The Association of Alcohol Consumption with Outcome of Pregnancy," *American Journal of Public Health* 73 (10): 1165-1168, 1983.

March of Dimes Foundation. "Will Drinking Hurt My Baby? [pamphlet] White Plains, NY: March of Dimes Birth Defects Foundation, 1986).

McIntire, Shelley A. "Annotated Bibliography on Fetal Alcohol Syndrome (FAS)," [unpublished] (Minneapolis: Minnesota Indian Women's Resource Center [1900 Chicago Avenue South, Minneapolis, MN 55404], 1986).

_____. "Bibliography on Children of Alcoholics," [unpublished] (Minneapolis: Minnesota Indian Women's Resource Center [1900 Chicago Avenue South, Minneapolis, MN 55404] 1986.

New York Times. "Birth Defects from Alcohol Persisting," 9/10/85.

New York Times. "Mother Who Gives Birth to Drug Addict Faces Felony Charge," 12/17/88.

New York Times. "Reports of New York Infants born with Drug Symptoms Up Sharply," 4/1/88.

Oppenheimer, Ingebor. "The Civil Liberties of the Unborn" (letter to the editor), *New York Times,* 10/23/86.

Osofsky J.: Neonatal Characteristics and Mother-Infant Interaction in Two Observational Situations. *Child Development* 1967; 47:1138-1147.

_____. Women, Drinking, and Pregnancy (New York: Metheun, 1986).

Sandor, G. G. S., D. F. Smith et al. "Cardiac Malformations in the Fetal Alcohol Syndrome," *Journal of Pediatrics* 98 (5): 771-773, 1981.

Sokol, R. J. "Alcohol and Abnormal Outcomes of Pregnancy," *Canadian Medical Association Journal* 125 (2): 143-148, 1981.

State of South Dakota. "House Bill 1310: For an Act To Require Alcoholic Beverage Licensees to Display Certain health Warnings," 61st Session, Legislative Assembly, Pierre, SD, 1986.

Streissguth, A. P. "Alcoholism and Pregnancy: An Overview and Update," *Journal of Substance and Alcohol Actions/Misuse* 4: 149-173, 1983.

_____. "Psychological Handicaps in Children with Fetal Alcohol Syndrome," *Annals of the New York Academy of Sciences,* 1976, 273: 140-145.

Taylor, Patricia. "It's Time To Put Warnings on Alcohol" (editorial), *New York Times,* 3/20/88.

USA Today. "Mom Accused of Fetus Neglect," 10/1/86.

U.S. News & World Report. "Alcohol, Poverty—The Killing Fields of Rosebud," pp. 52-53, 9/2/85.

U.S. News & World Report. "America's Richest, Poorest Counties," 93 (16): 18, 1982.

CHILDREN AND ALCOHOL

Alibrandi, Tom. **Young Alcoholics**, Minneapolis, MN: CompCare Publications, 1978.

Balcarzak, Ann M. **Hope for Young People with Alcoholic Parents.** Center City, MN: Hazelden Foundation, 1981.

Black, Claudia. **My Dad Loves Me, My Dad Has a Disease**. Newport Beach, CA: ACT, P.O. Box 8536, 1979.

Brooks, Cathleen. **The Secret Everyone Knows**. San Diego, CA: Operation Cork, 1981.

Figueroa, Ronny. **Pablito's Secret/El Secreto de Pablito.** Hollywood, FL: Health Communications, Inc., 1984.

Fox, Paula. **The Moonlight Man.** New York: Bradbury Press, 1986.

Heckler, JanEllen. **A Fragile Peace.** New York: G. P. Putnam's Sons, Inc., 1986.

Hornick-Beer, Edity Lynn. **A Teenager's Guide to Living With An Alcoholic Parent.** Center City, MN: Hazelden Educational Materials, 1984.

Jance, Judith A. **Welcome Home.** Edmonds, WA: Chas. Franklin Press, 1986.

Kenny, Kevin and Knoll, Helen. **Sometimes My Mom Drinks Too Much.** Milwaukee, WI: Raintree Publishers, 1980.

Porterfield, Kay Marie. **Coping With an Alcoholic Parent.** New York: The Rosen Publishing Group, 1985.

_____. **Familiar Strangers.** Center City, MN: Hazelden, 1984.

Seixas, Judith S. **Alcohol: What It Is, What It Does.** New York: Greenwillow Books, 1979.

_____. **Living With an Alcoholic Parent.** New York: Greenwillow Books. 1979.

Wheat, Patte. **You're Not Alone.** Chicago, IL: National Committee for Prevention of Child Abuse, 1985.

Families, Drugs and Alcohol

Biological/Genetic Factors in Alcoholism, Research Momograph 9. National Institute on Alcohol Abuse and Alcoholism. Drug Abuse and Mental Health Administration, U.S. Department of Health and Human Services. Rockville, MD. 1983.

Black, Claudia. **It Will Never Happen to Me.** MAC Printing and Publications Division, Denver, CO. 1982.

Califano, Joseph A. Jr., **Report on Drug Abuse and Alcoholism,** Warner Books, NY. 1982.

Coltoff, Philip and Luks, Allan. **Prevent Child Maltreatment: Begin With the Parent.** Children's Aid Society, NY. 1978.

Deutsch, Charles. **Broken Bottles, Broken Dreams.** Teachers College Press. Columbia University, NY. 1982.

_____. **Children of Alcoholics, Understanding and Helping.**
Hollywood, FL: Health Communications, Inc., 1983.

Devlin, Mark. **Stubborn Child—A Memoir.** New York:
Atheneum, 1985.

Dulfano. Celia. **Families, Alcoholism and Recovery—Ten
Stories.** Hazelden Foundation, Center City, MN. 1982.

Directory of National Resources for Children of Alcoholics,
Children of Alcoholics Foundation, Inc., NY, 1986.

Elkin, Michael. **Families Under the Influence: Changing
Alcoholic Patterns.** New York: W. W. Norton & Company,
1984.

Evans, David G. **Kids, Drugs, and the Law.** Center City, MN:
Hazelden Foundation, 1985.

**Fifth Special Report to the U.S. Congress on Alcohol and
Health.** National Institute on Alcohol Abuse and Alcoholism,
Alcohol, Drug and Mental Health Administration, U.S.
Department of Health and Human Services, December 1983.

Gravitz, Herbert L. and Bowden, Julie D. **Guide to Recovery.
A Book for Adult Children of Alcoholics.** Holmes Beach, FL:
Learning Publications, Inc., 1985.

Kaufman, Edward and Kaufmann, Pauline N. **Family Therapy
of Drug and Alcohol Abuse.** New York: Gardner Press, 1979.

Lawson, Gary, Peterson, James S., and Lawson, Ann.
**Alcoholism and the Family. A Guide to Treatment and
Prevention.** Rockville, MD: Aspen Systems Corporation, 1983.

Meryman, Richard. **Broken Promises. Mended Dreams.**
Boston: Little Brown and Company. 1984.

**Resource Directory of National Alcohol-Related
Associations, Agencies and Organizations,** National
Association of State Alcohol and Drug Abuse Directors,
Washington, D.C., 1985.

Pickens, Roy W. **Children of Alcoholics,** Center City, MN:
Hazelden Foundation, 1984.

Russell, Marcia, Henderson, Cynthia and Blume, Sheila.
Children of Alcoholics: A Review of the Literature. Children
of Alcoholics Foundation, Inc., NY, 1985.

Tower, Cynthia Crosson. **Child Abuse and Neglect: A Teacher's Handbook for Detection, Reporting and Classroom Management**, NEA Professional Library, National Education Association, Washington, D.C., 1984.

Valliant, George E. **The Natural History of Alcoholism.** Cambridge, MA: Harvard University Press, 1983.